Autophagy Mastery:

Follow the Autophagy Diet Healing Secrets That Many Men and Women Have Followed to Enhance Anti-Aging & Weight Loss for a Healthier Body, With Water Fasting & Intermittent Fasting!

By Elouisa Smith

Table of Contents

Autophagy Mastery:
Table of Contents
Introduction
Chapter 1: Putting Autophagy in Context
Chapter 2: The Three Kinds of Autophagy
Chapter 3: On a Molecular Level

    How Cells Get Energy
    Apoptosis
    The P62 Gene

Chapter 4: How to Control Autophagy in Your Body

    The Keto Diet and Autophagy
    Fasting Vs. Caloric Restriction
    Exercise
    Sleep
    Other Methods

Chapter 5: The Health Benefits of Mastering Autophagy

    The Detox
    The Short-Term Benefits
    The Long-Term Benefits

Chapter 6: Choose the Right Fast for You
Chapter 7: Diet and Supplements
Chapter 8: Helpful Facts about Autophagy

    The Glucose-Ketone Index
    When You Should Eat
    Try the Water Fast
    Common Mistakes
    Consistency
    Don't Neglect Exercise
    Eat Less Protein, Sometimes
    Protein Cycling

- Diversify Your Autophagy-Activating Methods
- The Benefits of Autophagy over Caloric Restriction
- Cardio vs. Resistance Training Exercise
- Autophagy Quotes

Chapter 9: How to Be Safe While Maximizing Autophagy

Chapter 10: The Mental Side

- Write It Down
- How Autophagy Changes Your Brain

Conclusion

Introduction

Congratulations on purchasing *Autophagy Mastery*, and thank you for doing so.

In this book, you'll learn how to detoxify your body by clearing out harmful chemicals at the cellular level. Scientific breakthroughs have been made in just the past couple of years that show the importance of autophagy in combating cancer and various age-related diseases. Follow our guidance and learn how to live healthily, long, and youthfully.

Maybe you have already tried a number of diets that claim to help you lose weight. Even if you did lose weight, you didn't keep it off. There is a good chance that not only did the diet not work in the long term, but it was also bad for your overall health.

It's time to be done with unhealthy diets that don't even work. In *Autophagy Mastery*, we'll talk about combining autophagy-inducing fasts with the ketogenic diet.

When you do both of these things — when you fast to activate autophagy and follow a ketogenic diet — you will surely lose weight. But you won't only do that — a keto diet combined with autophagy will heal your body.

We'll explain the science of how autophagy works, as well as how you can get the same health benefits that so many people are getting from these two lifestyle changes. We'll talk about autophagy first and foremost; activating autophagy is essential to keeping your body healthy and young.

Don't worry about getting overwhelmed with knowledge you haven't even heard of before. This book tells you everything you need to know about autophagy. If you read it from beginning to end, you'll be able to talk about autophagy for literally hours. Your friends and family will be skeptical at first, but since you'll have the scientific data and research to back it up, you'll make them want to learn more. And having people to fast with you makes it a lot easier!

Together your friends and family can join you on your journey, and everyone will better their lives.

There are plenty of books on this subject on the market, thanks again for choosing this one! Every effort was made to ensure it is full of as much useful information as possible; please enjoy!

Chapter 1: Putting Autophagy in Context

Before the dawn of agriculture, people did not expect food every day as a matter of fact. Human bodies were not used to eating several times every day. This meant that our bodies are more adapted to eating some days and fasting others than they are to eating every day.

Because of how much access to food we have in the developed world, autophagy has almost become a thing of the past. We almost never deprive ourselves of nutrients.

We live in a rapid modern world where we are always on. We are constantly putting things into our bodies with food, and putting information into our heads with digital media. The idea of cleansing sounds like it belongs to a different time because it certainly doesn't cohere with many ideals that people have today.

Christian De Duve coined the term autophagy in 1962 when the scientists in his lab noticed a strange organelle in yeast cells. It was later called the lysosome. Biologists have come a long way in understanding autophagy since then. The most exciting part about the newest findings are the implications for our health.

In the 1970s, biologists thought of autophagy as the lysosomes of our cells acting as garbage disposals, simply eliminating junk from our bodies. In 2016, Japanese cell biologist Yoshinori Ohsumi won the Nobel Prize in medicine or physiology for discovering the mechanisms of autophagy. First, Ohsumi discovered autophagy in a kind of cell called Baker's cells. His research showed that autophagy actually recycles materials in our bodies for reuse.

Ohsumi defined autophagy as the cell's process of destroying content to make room for more cells, fight microbes and pathogens, generate materials for new cells, and reuse these materials for new components.

He decided to study autophagy when the number of scientists focusing on it was very small, but ever since his ground-breaking discoveries that earned him the Nobel Prize, many scientists have become interested in autophagy.

In an interview, Ohsumi has said autophagy is a means of cell recycling. Cell recycling happens when nutrients are scarce, and autophagy kicks in to destroy old machinery to make new machinery. Ohsumi's study showed us how autophagy takes center stage in cell recycling. It is pretty surprising that most scientists had not paid much attention to autophagy before, because now we understand that it is an essential process in all living things.

Without autophagy, cells could not go through cell recycling, and they would simply die after their organelles no longer worked, or when they were taken over by foreign invaders. We know that autophagy is a way you can make your cells last longer and stay like younger cells.

Much of our new understanding of autophagy can be credited to Ohsumi. His discovery of the role of autophagy in cell recycling is how we know about autophagy's connection to Parkinson's and Alzheimer's. These diseases have turned out to result from a mutation in an autophagy gene.

Autophagy is how our cells survive under stress. Understanding autophagy helps us understand how our bodies react to starvation, stress, and infection. It was this implication of autophagy that the Nobel Assembly credited to Ohsumi's award of the Nobel Prize.

There is no doubt that Ohsumi's work will be credited as the necessary precursor to research that will find cures in the future. Ohsumi's research has paved the way for looking for cures, but until then, we can use our knowledge of the importance of autophagy to make activating it a part of our routine.

Since our DNA degrades as we age, mutations like these are more common in older adults. This makes it all the more important to initiate autophagy in your body, no matter your age.

Besides the research showing the benefits of fasting-induced autophagy for cancer patients going through chemotherapy, the most recent studies are on the effects of different drugs on autophagy and the resulting slowing of cancer cell growth.

Drugs that stimulate autophagy have proved to slow the growth of cancer cells for neuroblastoma. The cancer cells were put in a petri dish with the drug rabocymin and showed inhibited growth compared to cancer cells without the drug.

The non-cancer cells in the dish were even able to better destroy the cancer cells, thanks to the autophagy-boosting drug. The neuroblastoma cancer cell study was just one of many similar clinical trials that have been done in recent years.

More work needs to be done in this area before it can truly save people's lives, but it is still an exciting time to be alive with all the advancements being made.

It is very important for autophagy to break down the damaged organelles in your cells because, at a certain point, they require more energy to keep running than they are worth in function. It makes more sense for the cell to go through autophagy and break down these organelles and make new ones.

Autophagy is stimulated by stress, but you don't want chronic stress. You want acute stress. Acute stress is a kind of stress that happens only over a short period of time — the kind that comes from fasting and exercise.

Chapter 2: The Three Kinds of Autophagy

The three kinds of autophagy are microautophagy, macroautophagy, and chaperone-mediated autophagy. All cells have lysosomes that engage in microautophagy on their own, pulling in damaged organelles and other materials for breakdown. The purpose of microautophagy is for membrane homeostasis, cell survival, and to maintain organelle size. In the lysosome, enzymes are released that attack the contents. These contents are used for amino acids, glucose, fatty acids, and more.

All cells go through microautophagy. Lysosomes fuse with damaged organelles to destroy and use them for parts for new organelles. This is all part of the essential cell cycle that Ohsumi uncovered in his Nobel prize-winning research.

Macroautophagy happens in only specialized cells; a vesicle called the autophagosome goes outside the cell to transport materials in the cytoplasm to the lysosome for breakdown. The process of transporting cargo into the lysosome is called sequestration. In macroautophagy, the lysosome does not break down the materials, but rather the autophagosome. The autophagosome binds with the lysosome and breaks down the components inside.

Macroautophagy is also known as phagocytosis. Only specialized cells, such as white blood cells, undergo this kind of autophagy. When these cells encounter a large particle, they extend the autophagosome to engulf it, and then the autophagosome merges with the lysosome to break it down for reusable parts.

There are also kinds of macroautophagy that are organelle-specific. They are mitophagy, pexophagy, and ribophagy. These types remove damaged organelles.

Chaperone-mediated autophagy is the newest kind we know of: in it, specialized proteins work with the lysosome to help transport specific particles to the lysosome. Chaperone-mediated autophagy has been shown to be very important in several physiological processes such as DNA repair, metabolism, and the regulation of glucose.

The process of chaperone-mediated autophagy is similar to that of microautophagy, but instead of degrading any materials in the cells that aren't helping it function, it degrades specific cytosol components. Your cells know which components to degrade with chaperone-mediated autophagy because of the direction they receive from their genes.

The most recent breakthroughs in research tell us that chaperone-mediated autophagy is the most important type of autophagy when it comes to age-related illness. Scientists have discovered a clear link between diseases like cancer and the degeneration of the brain.

This is because, as we age, the cellular components necessary for this more elaborate type of autophagy degrade. As a result, microbes and other toxins can infiltrate the cells with less resistance, and the discarded proteins in your cells can build up and lead to neurodegenerative diseases like Alzheimer's and Parkinson's.

But you don't have to accept this as an inevitable result of aging. You can maximize the benefits of autophagy naturally by following the instructions in this book. We'll tell you all the practical knowledge you will ever need to have to get the most out of autophagy.

Chaperone-mediated autophagy uses chaperone proteins to guide proteins across the membrane of the lysosome. There, the targeted proteins are digested. This is the most advanced form of autophagy we know of, and as a result, we know the least about it. But it does show great promise for the prevention of curing of age-related diseases.

Chaperone-mediated autophagy is a great example of how autophagy is always happening through your body in different places at different times. It is active in your kidney, liver, and heart at different times, for example. When it comes to chaperone-mediated autophagy, it is not a question of whether it is happening, but where.

Your cells will switch to this special kind of autophagy after about ten hours of fasting and starvation. It reaches a plateau of activation within about 36 hours, and it can stay at this level for three days.

While all forms of autophagy will remove, reuse, and recycle dysfunctional proteins, chaperone-mediated autophagy is responsible for the selective removal of dysfunctional proteins.

The specialized protein at the surface of the lysosome in chaperone-mediated autophagy is called LAMP-2A, which stands for lysosome associated membrane protein. Studies on mice demonstrated that when we preserve this protein through the lifespans of mice, they lived longer and were healthier.

In more recent studies, scientists modulated chaperone-mediated autophagy on transgenic mouse models in vivo, and they found that this kind of autophagy can regulate many cell functions besides breaking down protein. When chaperone-mediated autophagy breaks down the right proteins at the right times, it helps with lipid and glucose metabolism, cellular reprogramming, and even DNA repair. Since damaged DNA can lead to many age-related diseases, scientists are especially interested in this function of chaperone-mediated autophagy.

In the neurodegenerative disease Parkinson's, scientists have shown defects in the activity of chaperone-mediated autophagy. The defect occurs because toxic proteins bind to LAMP-2A with abnormal affinity, which causes clogging in the cells.

You may have accumulated a lot of protein build-ups in your cells over time, but we'll tell you the best ways to activate autophagy, getting your cells to clean them up and recycle them.

If you're looking to prevent the onset of disease as you age, autophagy will help accomplish this, too. Autophagy improves the body's immune function along with several other biofactors, and when you activate it, you help prevent infections that cause cancer and other diseases.

Chapter 3: On a Molecular Level

Even though they are microscopic, cells make everything you do possible. One of the most salient effects of aging is cell damage. The organelles in the cells of older adults are less effective. Autophagy minimizes the effects of aging on your cellular biology. Doing this decreases the effects of aging and makes you live longer.

If you don't start a new routine of activating autophagy, your cells will not get rid of waste and toxins nearly as well, and as a result, your cells won't function as well. This will lead to weight gain, worse skin, increased inflammation, less energy, and age-related disease. Fasting and learning healthier habits will decrease the effects of aging by keeping your cells youthful.

Multiple genes and proteins come into play at the various stages of autophagy, but the practical knowledge you need to have is very straightforward.

First, you want to know how you would explain autophagy to someone in a few sentences. The word autophagy is made of two parts with Greek origins: "auto" means "self," and "phagy" means "to eat." And that's precisely what autophagy is. When your cells go through autophagy, they eat parts of themselves that you might call junk.

Your cells' damaged mitochondria don't function as well, so your cells eat them up and use the parts to build new, healthy mitochondria. The proteins that your cells use become useless over time, and end up simply taking up space and doing nothing.

The mitochondria may be the most important part of the cell. As the powerhouse, it produces energy for the entire cell. A healthy mitochondria affects the whole cell positively. Healthy mitochondria are what best prevent neurodegenerative diseases such as Alzheimer's and Parkinson's.

The metaphor of car repair is fitting here. If your car was broken down and fixing it wasn't worth the cost, you wouldn't be able to sell it. You wouldn't let it stay in your yard for years and years, either. It would be an ugly thing to look at for you and passersby.

You would do one of two things. If you aren't mechanically gifted, you would find someone who would buy it for parts at a good rate. If you know how a car works, you would take it apart yourself and use the parts for a new car.

Your cells do the same thing. When the toxins start to pile up and make a mess, they clean them out and make use of them.

Autophagy is when your cells are starved of nutrients, so they feed on nutrients that are already present in your body. Autophagy is the reason that we humans are able to survive for three weeks without food. You and your cells continue to survive because your cells use the nutrients that are already inside the tiny crevasses of their cytoplasm.

The body requires about a hundred grams of protein every day. You might be surprised to hear that only about a third of this protein comes from the food you eat. The rest of the protein comes from autophagy. Autophagy breaks down the protein in your body for reuse; this is where most of your protein comes from.

Your cells already have build-ups of damaged proteins, dysfunctional organelles, and foreign toxins. These accumulate just by living life. Every plant and animal undergoes autophagy when the cells undergo stress or starvation.

As we discussed, the finer details of autophagy on the molecular level are still being studied in the lab, but we know the fundamental steps that make it up. The most important types of autophagy from the perspective of your health are macroautophagy and chaperone-mediated autophagy.

A special vesicle called the autophagosome goes outside the cell and traps materials inside its double membrane. Then, it returns to the cell and merges with a vacuole called the lysosome (the cell stomach). From there, the autophagosome breaks down the pathogens, damaged organelles, or misfolded proteins the same way it does in any type of autophagy.

We will go into detail on the lifestyle changes that will activate and maximize autophagy, but it is still good to know some of the inner workings of the genes that activate it at the lowest level of every cell.

Your cells carry their own DNA and genes. Your genes are able to detect small changes in your cells — when they detect a low amount of nutrients, they activate autophagy, getting your proteins to perform the necessary functions to do so.

Among the many genes involved in autophagy, ATG is the most important. ATG isn't an acronym; instead, it is supposed to look like the word "AuTophaGy" because it is the essential autophagy-related gene. The gene ATG and the protein chain VPS-34 are essential for the regulation and stimulation of autophagy.

Research shows that manipulating the VPS-34 protein chain network may benefit scientists looking for a way to fight disease. This is because many age-related diseases can be traced back to the degradation of the systems that are essential to autophagy. Once scientists figure out how to manipulate ATG and VPS-34 at a fine level and inevitably change medicine and aging, simply know that ATG and VPS-34 are the main gene and protein chain to be aware of. You may also want to know about the gene HIF-1A, which starts hypoxia in your cells when they undergo autophagy.

The accumulation of cellular garbage hinders your healthy functioning at the microscopic level. Autophagy's purpose is to maintain homeostasis in your cells by keeping your proteins at healthy levels and keeping out harmful toxins. It is your body's natural process of cleaning all of this out of your system and repurposing it for better use.

There is a consensus among scientists that a lack of autophagy can lead to buildups of proteins in brain cells that lead to neurodegenerative diseases, which we have established. But there is a similar phenomenon with diabetes as well.

The problem of accumulating misfolded proteins is not limited to cells in the brain. When cells in any part of your body accumulate a lot of misfolded proteins because they hardly go through autophagy, these proteins clump together to form what are known as amyloid deposits.

There is a common misconception that autophagy only helps fight disease because it fights pathogens and toxins that come from the outside of the cell. While it's true that autophagy fights infections by trapping toxic invaders in the lysosome and breaking them down for usable parts (talk about brutal!), autophagy also fights against disease by preventing the accumulation of toxins from within the cell.

When your cells have too many useless organelles and proteins that no longer perform a function in the cell, they eventually become toxic, leading to the cells prematurely dying. Ideally, you induce autophagy often so that your cells clean out these toxic proteins and organelles. This way, your cells live longer and stay healthy.

That's where your part in this comes in. Cells don't have a will of their own to clean up their mess. If you want them to clean their room, so to speak, you have to make them do it.

You make your cells undergo autophagy by starving them of the nutrients from the foods you eat. In our modern world, we spoil our cells by feeding them multiple times every day. As a result, they don't keep things tidy and running smoothly.

But your cells need nutrients to keep going. That's why when you stop eating, they take care of the damaged organelles and proteins and use them for food. This happens in cells all over your body, detoxifying your system, and leaving you feeling great.

The pores in your skin clear up, the higher efficiency of unclogged cells gives you more energy, and best of all, you lose weight. You get all these benefits without the health risks of diets that have no basis in science. People who change their lifestyles around fasting and inducing autophagy see these results in as little as two weeks.

Mastering autophagy comes down to refining a balance between the activation of two enzymes: mTOR and AMPK. The enzyme mTOR is activated when you eat, that is, when you have significant levels of glucose in your body.

AMPK is the opposite: it activates when you don't eat. When your cell energy is low, it activates glucose, fatty acid uptake, and oxidation. When your energy is low, AMPK starts the process of autophagy.

When you don't eat, your glucose goes down, and a hormone called glucagon goes up. If you have enough glucose in your body, your cells consume the nutrients you eat. Alternatively, when you have high levels of glucagon, autophagy is activated.

You can look at the activation of AMPK as what stimulates autophagy and what activates catabolism. You can look at the activation of mTOR (through eating) as what stops autophagy and activates anabolism.

Catabolism is the breakdown of complex molecules in living things to form simpler ones, a process that requires energy. You should associate catabolism with an increase in glucagon, the hormone that ultimately initiates autophagy.

The activation of mTOR (caused by the increase of glucose) starts the process of anabolism. Anabolism is the synthesis of molecules in living things from simpler molecules to more complex ones, a process that also requires energy.

On the molecular level, anabolism and catabolism are important parts of autophagy. When the lysosome and autophagosome break down cell components into usable materials, this is catabolism. Your cells need to change the complex composition of the molecules they eat into simpler molecules so they can change them into something else. In the stage of autophagy, where these simple molecules are built into new organelles, this is anabolism.

Your cells need both anabolism and catabolism to stay healthy. These opposite but equally necessary processes further emphasize the importance of balance in autophagy. Eat on your feasting days so your cells can make something out of the broken-down parts through anabolism; fast on your fasting days so your cells can break down garbage into simpler molecules through catabolism.

How Cells Get Energy

You have probably heard of the molecule ATP before. ATP stands for adenosine triphosphate, and it is the main source of energy in cells. Whether your body's cells get energy from autophagy or the processing of nutrients, the end product is still energy generated from the breakdown of ATP.

Everything you do requires energy. You even require energy to break down the food that gives you energy. You require energy to use your muscles, have thoughts, sleep, and replicate your cells' DNA.

ATP stands for adenosine triphosphate. This molecule is vital to your metabolism. Other molecules called respiratory complex fill this same role, but ATP is more abundant and more important. You can find all the beautiful details of the process of ATP phosphorylation from other sources: it is the process that gives us energy and makes all life possible. This book just wants you to understand it well enough to take control of it.

Essentially, your cells break down adenosine triphosphate (ATP) into adenosine diphosphate (ADP). This releases the energy stored in the binding of that extra phosphate. The energy you get from ATP is how your body can run. Your cells are in a constant cycle of converting ATP into ADP and back into ATP again.

Turning ADP back into ATP requires food as well as oxygen. Animals and plants alike go through this process of converting ATP into ADP and back again. Animals change ADP back to ATP through the process of oxidation, and plants change ADP to ATP through carbon dioxide in photosynthesis.

At any given moment, your body only has eight ounces of ATP — but every single day, it produces an equivalent of 175 pounds of

ATP. This is approximately the weight of an average human. This is 200 septillion ATP molecules or 2 followed by twenty-six zeroes.

Producing your entire body weight in ADP every single day sounds like an exhausting process, but a healthy body does it without disrupting any other processes.

When you age, you still have to break down the nutrients you get from food. The more food you metabolize, the more energy you burn. Over the course of your lifetime, this gradually erodes your body and cells. As a result, they become less able to break down ATP over time.

If you eat less, your cells will metabolize less and take longer to erode. They end up being more resilient later in life because they experienced less wear and tear. This is the principle idea of caloric restriction, which has been shown to increase lifespan in animals and health in humans. The jury is still out on whether caloric restriction increases lifespan for humans.

Alternatively to caloric restriction, autophagy is scientifically proven to be important to age-related illness, so we are better off stimulating autophagy and still getting fewer calories by fasting.

Apoptosis

Autophagy is also a means of reusing the parts left behind from dead cells. Cells either die from trauma, lack of nutrients, or they go through a planned process of cell death. There are many terms for the planned death of a cell: autophagic cell death, programmed cell death, or apoptosis. Apoptosis is usually done to maintain homeostasis with the rest of the tissue of which the cell forms a part.

If a cell is damaged or it just isn't necessary for the function of the surrounding tissue, it may go through apoptosis. Surrounding cells can break down the dead cell and use it for materials. It may seem harsh, but sometimes this is a good way for your body to clean itself and maintain proper efficiency.

We should be very aware of the difference between autophagy and apoptosis because people tend to get them confused. Apoptosis is the highly controlled process of programmed cell death. Necrosis is when a cell dies because of trauma, infection, or lack of nutrients — apoptosis is different because the death is programmed. Sometimes this is done to make room for more tissue. It can also be done for self-destruction because the cell recognizes that it is harming the body. If the cell is cancerous, it may initiate apoptosis.

It is always good to be aware of the different biological processes happening in our body, but you should know that apoptosis and autophagy are very different. This matters because when people hear that autophagy means "self-eating," they sometimes get confused and think they are eating other cells, or eating themselves as in self-destruction in the process of apoptosis.

If you use the term "self-eating" when thinking about autophagy, add "self-renewal" after it. This will save a lot of confusion.

The P62 Gene

The link between autophagy and the P62 gene tells a fascinating story about human evolution. The P62 gene has been credited to the human lifespan being as long as it is, due to our superior response to acute biological stress.

But humans did not always have this gene. We evolved to have it over time.

Since we have the P62 gene, whenever the body detects metabolic byproducts that cause cell damage, the P62 gene induces autophagy to clean the byproducts out.

The P62 gene is the most famous and well understood among autophagy researchers, but we are talking about it to make a point that many genes are in play in autophagy, all with different purposes. It's true the enzyme AMPK activates autophagy, but it is far from the only player. There are many players like the P62 gene that take part.

When scientists gave fruit flies the P62 gene, they survived longer in stressful conditions. The fact that even a fruit fly can benefit from this human autophagy gene shows how powerful it really is.

Chapter 4: How to Control Autophagy in Your Body

Cells form systems in their trillions. They generate energy in their mitochondria and communicate with one another. Even though there are always some who are going through autophagy, there is a huge difference between a few hundred thousand going through autophagy, millions of cells going through autophagy, or ten of billions of cells going through autophagy. If you have this book, I suspect you want the last one to happen so you can keep your body as clean and healthy as possible.

Young cells do their jobs with near perfection. Hardly anyone has to think about their health when they are young for this reason. Cells wear and tear as you age, but you don't have to accept this as a fact of life. They will degrade, but if you allow your cells to heal themselves, they will not degrade nearly as much. Stimulating autophagy is an effective way to put a stopper on aging.

Healthier cells mean a healthier body. Your cells will automatically eat some of their toxins and do some of the work on their own, but it is not nearly as effective as when you activate it for longer periods of time through the methods in this book.

The frustrating thing about stimulating autophagy as we get older is that since our cells have degraded over time, not only are they are less able to perform their normal functions, but they are also less able to perform autophagy. This is an irritating fact to deal with since we want to induce autophagy in order to improve the health of our cells.

The good news is that your autophagy will still clean out your cells no matter your age and every toxin they remove in the process will help them the next time you activate autophagy.

This is part of the reason that I strongly emphasize the importance of consistency when it comes to autophagy. You will make great strides in your body when you do your first fast; your body will rid itself of countless toxins and make itself healthier.

But consistency matters because if you follow up with another fast after a few days of eating, your cells will be better able to clean themselves through autophagy than the first time.

Autophagy is not something that you can expect to help you if you only fast once a year. The long-term benefits of such an infrequent fast are not backed up by the research, but the effects of regular fasting are.

Don't fast a few times a year and expect it to do your health any significant good in the long term. You will probably feel amazing after your first fast, but if you don't fast for another few months after, you pretty much brought your body back to square one. It will take time to get into a habit of regularly fasting, but once you have, the benefits will come in how you feel.

After learning the science of autophagy from the last chapter, you can see why fasting is an essential part of controlling it in your body. However, we want you to be aware of the important balance you must strike when controlling autophagy. One way to go about this healthily is to alternate between days of fasting and days of eating autophagy-enhancing foods.

You need a rich diet of nutrient-rich foods to feed your cells on your feasting days, and you need to consume nothing but water on your fasting days to activate autophagy and clear out toxins and junk from your body.

Sometimes when people learn about autophagy and start getting interested in it, they get a false idea that autophagy is either "on" or "off." In reality, autophagy is happening in your body at all times in different cells across your organs. It's not so black and white as "off" or "on."

When I say that following the practices in the book will activate autophagy, it doesn't mean none of your cells were undergoing autophagy and suddenly will when you fast and exercise. The truth is a matter of scale.

At this very moment, there are cells in your body going through autophagy, but if you lifted weights earlier, many more cells would be going through autophagy. If you were 24 hours into a fast and you had just exercised, even more, cells would be going through autophagy.

You want to go beyond the autophagy that happens in your body today and get the most out of this natural process. This is what the practices in the book are meant to accomplish. If you didn't make any changes after reading this book, of course, autophagy would still happen in your body, but much less. The longer your body's cells undergo autophagy, the more time they have to clear out toxins by breaking them down for energy.

The Keto Diet and Autophagy

The keto diet is another way to increase autophagy in your body. We recommend that you get the greatest possible benefit by combining fasting and the keto diet, but your body and health are ultimately up to you.

To burn glucose, your body uses carbohydrates. If you follow the keto diet and eat healthy fats and fewer carbs, the power of autophagy increases. The same thing happens when you fast, but with a diet rich in healthy fats, you also get the added benefits of unsaturated fats. In the Diet and Supplements chapters, I'll discuss how a diet filled with healthy fasts will help to boost autophagy.

Fasting Vs. Caloric Restriction

If you are constantly eating with no breaks of fasting, you are not giving your cells time to repair from the damage of toxins that accumulate while eating. Research shows that intermittent fasting promotes higher energy levels, the increase of fat-burning, and also decreases your risk of diabetes and heart disease. These benefits are all thanks to the stimulation of autophagy through the starvation of your cells.

Recall that autophagy is induced in your cells because of stress. Stress can come in the form of starvation, exercise, and rapidly changing the temperature of your environment. Stress means something different to your cells than it does to you. You don't feel tired while you're sleeping, but even without fasting, our cells go through some level of autophagy because of the stress of not having nutrients for eight hours.

Fasting is one of the most effective methods of activating autophagy according to the research, but there are several ways to activate it. Incorporating many of them into your life will net you the most health benefit.

When you fast, your cells need to undergo autophagy in order to get energy. We already went over how the lysosome and autophagosome break down toxins and convert them into usable materials, but this process of "eating" also generates energy for the cell. In autophagy, the process of breaking down ATP for energy happens with the toxins in your cells instead of with the foods you eat.

In a diet, you limit the foods you eat, but you are still eating. When you fast, you go through periods of time without eating at all. Fasting is what will stimulate high levels of autophagy for long periods of time.

About fifteen years ago, the idea of caloric restriction gained a lot of attention and popularity among people who wanted to be healthier, lose weight, and live longer. There were, in fact, studies showing that mammals who restricted their consumption by 10% saw an increase in lifespan. They also saw improvement in biomarkers of health, such as blood pressure and inflammation.

The theory of caloric restriction to improve health certainly had its merits, but autophagy edges it out in all respects. For one, if you fast every other day and eat healthy foods on the days you aren't fasting, you are already restricting your calorie intake significantly.

That means you are getting the same benefits of caloric restriction as well as benefiting from increased autophagy.

There is also the simple fact that caloric restriction never got the same scientific backing as autophagy. While biologists still have more to learn about autophagy, we know for a fact that autophagy plays a big role in aging and age-related illnesses.

If you make inducing autophagy a focus in your life, you will get the potential benefits of caloric restriction while also forcing your cells to detoxify your body on your fasting days. You get the best of both worlds.

If you think fasting for just 12 hours won't make a difference, know that the constantly growing research on autophagy says you are wrong. One study showed that decreasing your feeding window just by a tiny few hours had positive effects on autophagy.

Since you are reading this book, you are surely looking to boost your autophagy more than it was boosted from this small change. But what you should take away from this study is that every little change you make that improves your health will make a big difference, especially when autophagy is concerned.

One famous study looked at one group of rats that had a high-fat diet, but could only eat during 8 hours of the day (so they fasted for 16 hours). The other group had the same diet but could eat whenever they wanted to. The fasting group had fewer health problems than the group that did not fast.

Another study followed ten-month-old mice that went without food twice a week in order to trigger autophagy. After six weeks, the mice that did the fast gained weight at the same rate as the non-fasting mice. But when all the mice were 24 months old, the cells in their immune systems were studied, and the fasting mice were shown to have more youthful immune systems than the non-fasting mice.

One of the researchers made a point that the fur of the fasting mice was also shinier and healthier. These fasting mice were healthier in many ways, just as we humans can be if we induce autophagy through fasting and exercise.

Exercise

So far, we have only talked about fasting and dieting to induce autophagy. But there is an equally important factor that people usually dread: exercise. Studies have shown that people who fasted for 36 hours underwent less autophagy than people who did resistance training for short 20-minute sessions.

When hearing of this study, remember that it's the level of autophagy that we are always concerned with. Autophagy is not "off" or "on." Rather, it happens at different degrees, from maintenance mode to greater and greater degrees of advanced autophagy. Fasting will undoubtedly put you in advanced autophagy, but it is possible that exercise will get you even more.

Don't limit yourself by reading this as "Fasting is pointless, and I should only exercise." Read it as more opportunity for autophagy optimization. You have so many options for activating and enhancing autophagy; if you want to get as much out of it as possible, you should try to pull out all the stops by fasting, dieting, and exercising.

Autophagy clears up the damage to cells that happens as a result of exercise. When your cells are repaired, your energy levels are increased.

When autophagy was induced with exercise, there were no positive results in the skeletal muscle fibers. But when autophagy was induced with fasting, the mice were able to prevent the degeneration of their muscle fibers and the accumulation of damaged organelles.

Basically, this showed that fasting could contribute to the autophagy-inducing effects of exercise. It is beneficial to maintain the homeostasis of our muscles during exercise. Fasting, along with exercise, was especially helpful for the regeneration of collagen in skin cells.

It is also yet another study that shows how exercise and fasting can give more benefits to autophagy depending on the situation, which is why we keep reminding you not to pick one or the other. Choose both.

It is educational, if not surprising, to note this fact: in a study of fasting that measured the autophagy of trained athletes against non-athletes, the athletes saw much greater autophagy than the other group.

You might think this is because athletes are predisposed to having better overall health, but when you look at the research on how much exercise activates autophagy, it seems probable that the active lifestyles of the athletes were a key factor in their increased autophagy.

Sleep

Sleep is the most mysterious element of autophagy activation because scientists still do not understand what it is for. Did you know that lying down while awake only saves 100 more calories than sleeping? This suggests that the purpose of sleep has more to do with the brain than the body.

Sleep itself won't stimulate autophagy as well as these other methods, but don't get the wrong idea — you will require eight hours of high-quality sleep every night if you want to get the most out of all of your autophagy-boosting methods.

As you sleep, your body repairs damage and autophagy reaches its highest point in the day. Because you are doing nothing but sleeping, this allows your body to expend much more energy to these tasks.

The flip side is also true regarding autophagy and sleep: your body undergoes much more autophagy in your sleep, but if you are deprived of sleep, much less autophagy will happen in your body.

Being tired itself can increase inflammation, so be sure to get plenty of sleep. The quality of your sleep is more important than how long you sleep.

It is harder for your body to keep up with autophagy and the growth of new cells if you do not keep a regular circadian rhythm. Be sure not to go outside this rhythm so your body can keep up.

Being deprived of sleep will also make you more likely to suffer from metabolic inflexibility, lack of self-control, brain fog, and cravings.

While we're on the topic of sleep, we have to consider our circadian rhythms. Since you sleep for eight hours, you should be eating at maximum for eight hours a day. This balance between consumption and digestion is another way to think about autophagy. Whenever you put things into your body, you need to take an equal amount of time to cleanse your body.

Other Methods

Now we will touch on some other methods of activating autophagy. These methods will give you a shorter-lasting effect than fasting and following the keto diet, but they are still worth noting if you want to detoxify your body as much as possible.

You can use a sauna to activate autophagy. When you sweat from the heat of the sauna, this will put stress on your cells, which you recall is always what triggers autophagy. Just be sure to follow the standard health guidelines for using saunas, and you will have this extra way to detoxify.

If you are able to visit a sauna, this is another great way to activate autophagy. It strengthens your immune system, detoxifies your body, lowers your heart rate, and improves blood circulation. These effects are all due to the heat stress that saunas put on your cells, triggering AMPK, and putting your cells in advanced autophagy.

The next method may seem unusual. You can put stress on your cells (and induce autophagy) by quickly changing the temperature of your environment. If it's cold outside, you can spend a couple of minutes outside and then run back inside to heat back up. You can also take a cold shower for a bit, and then switch the water to hot (be very careful not to burn yourself if you try this!).

Acupuncture will put stress on your body and induce autophagy.

Chapter 5: The Health Benefits of Mastering Autophagy

The Detox

I hope that by now, this book has made you think about detox in a new way. A lot of "juice diets" claim to detoxify you by consuming as much kale as humanly possible, but there is no real evidence to support these proclaimed health benefits.

In contrast, autophagy happens naturally in your body, whether you know about it or not. Stimulating it does not do something new for your body; when you boost and stimulate autophagy, you are simply making the most out of an intracellular process that all living things go through.

Autophagy detoxified your body long before any of these juice diets even existed, and autophagy will detoxify you more than they ever will.

The Short-Term Benefits

One of the ways you can increase the autophagy in your body is by tweaking your diet. We'll go over the foods containing chemicals that stimulate the proteins and genes that play a role in autophagy.

Changing your diet alone won't unleash the full power of autophagy, but it will still make a difference — for your skin in particular. It will make the fastest difference on the epidermis, the outer layer of your skin. Autophagy helps to clean out the pores in your skin, giving you shinier, more youthful skin.

The way this works is twofold. Autophagy cleans toxins out of your skin by breaking them down, but it also improves the overall condition of your skin cells, which helps them produce more of a protein called collagen.

If you want to make your skin look clearer, controlling your collagen is the way to go. Your collagen is responsible for making skin elastic and durable. As we age, our skin cells produce less collagen because our cells lose the efficiency they once had. The parts of our cells get crowded out by the damaged proteins and damaged organelles that autophagy cleans out. This means that not only does autophagy by cleaning out this excess material, but it improves the efficiency of your cells so they can produce more collagen.

Revitalizing your skin cells isn't the only way autophagy slows aging. If you get into a habit of regularly initiating autophagy in your body, autophagy will stave off cancer and neurodegeneration.

Skin is important because it protects you from UV rays and diseases. The breakdown of collagen leads to wrinkles; it can be caused by sun exposure and mere aging. The cells in your skin are replaced about every thirty days. Your skin goes through a continual process of renewal.

Skin care protects only cover the outer surface of your skin with what is basically a coat of paint. In the long term, these products can lead to the inflammation of the skin, burning, and acne. If you are serious about keeping healthy skin, you should try to drink 8-10 glasses of water a day.

To understand why autophagy does such a great job of keeping your skin healthy, you'll want to understand why skin ages in the first place.

Your skin is made of cells called fibroblasts that create a protein known as collagen. Collagen acts as connective tissue in many parts of your body. The skin is where collagen is most prevalent since it is your largest organ.

When we get older, our fibroblasts produce less collagen, making your skin lose the elasticity it once had. Our fibroblasts produce less collagen because we have fewer autophagosomes when we get older, so these cells are less able to recycle their components to create more collagen. With age also comes more cellular stress and degradation as a whole due to your time alive, which also reduces autophagy's ability to work as well as it used to.

But rather than take this as a fact of life, you should be motivated to stimulate autophagy to the greatest extent possible.

Stimulating autophagy makes your fibroblasts healthier and more efficient, helping them produce more collagen. The result is clearer, tighter, and more youthful skin.

After you have gone some time fasting, the first thing you should check to see the progress of autophagy is your skin. If you have clear skin with a good tone, then autophagy is already doing its work on you. This is more likely than not because of a difference in skin tone, and weight are the first things people tend to notice after practicing autophagy-activating lifestyles.

You won't be able to know for sure if it was the autophagy or some other factors, but if you practice the habits in this book for a few months and notice improved skin tone, it is very probable that you should credit autophagy to the difference.

We should really be more concerned about the health benefits of autophagy rather than the cosmetic benefits such as on the skin and on weight. But there is nothing wrong with appreciating these changes as a bonus.

The main issue with focusing too much on the "vain" side of autophagy is that it might make you stop your autophagy-boosting habits once you have the results you want. As we make clear throughout the book, autophagy is not something that is one-and-done. If you don't consistently practice these techniques, the benefits will not last.

But perhaps the thing people hate most about aging is the decreased elasticity of the skin. This concern is why the anti-aging industry is worth billions of dollars. When it comes to skin care, the great thing about autophagy is that it already happens naturally in your body. Even better is that you have a great degree of control over autophagy.

Sometimes people are concerned about fasting or dieting to lose weight because they are worried about having loose skin afterward.

But since fasting activates autophagy and improves the health of your skin, loose skin is less of an issue when you lose weight.

Compared to people who just diet, people who fast report having less loose skin after losing weight. Not only is their skin healthier, but it is tighter after fasting. If you combine a consistent habit of fasting with regular exercise, autophagy will be even more effective, and your skin will be even tighter than without exercise.

"Skin curtain" is the term for the excess skin you might have after losing weight. If you lose weight without fasting to induce autophagy, skin curtains are a very common occurrence.

Your skin cells eventually die when they no longer function properly. You can get your healthy cells to stay youthful longer through autophagy; they will take the damaged organelles from the bad cells and recycle them to make new parts.

Clearing out your skin cells through autophagy will give your skin a brighter tone and a new glow. When you activate autophagy, you are cleaning out toxins that make it harder for you to gain weight, so you will notice significant weight loss, as well. It also reduces inflammation in your body, greatly reducing your risk of all related diseases.

The benefits of improved skin and weight loss are just the ones you get in the short term. Ever since Ohsumi's Nobel prize-winning research on the health implications of autophagy, we also know the long-term benefits of inducing autophagy.

The Long-Term Benefits

Even if autophagy doesn't suppress tumors, we know for sure that it promotes the survival of cells during spontaneous and induced nutrient stress. However, it is widely accepted that cases of Alzheimer's, Huntington's, Parkinson's disease, and certain heart diseases could be prevented by the healing factor of autophagy. This is because autophagy promotes cell viability and survival.

Until the last few years, scientists didn't think of autophagy as being such a big player in these diseases. We now know that autophagy is a powerful game-changer in the progression of disease.

The research has made clear that the mutation or damage of autophagy-related genes leads to age-related illnesses. These illnesses include cancer, neuropathies, heart disease, autoimmune disease, and other conditions. The jury is still out on whether autophagy suppresses tumors, but the important thing is that we prevent tumors in the first place with autophagy. We do this by keeping our cells clean and healthy, allowing them to fight off disease.

You see, amyloid deposits in the arteries of people with diabetes. Instead of allowing these proteins to accumulate and cause disease, you can clean them up with autophagy.

The scientific consensus is that autophagy plays a key role in clearing out toxic proteins that lead to diseases like Alzheimer's and Parkinson's. Autophagy lowers your blood pressure and improves autoimmune function. When you lose weight, it helps prevent all the risks associated with obesity. Autophagy is the best way to increase your lifespan, make you healthier, and look younger.

Autophagy research on cancer patients undergoing chemotherapy has shown promising results as well. Scientists had one group of people go through a fast while they went through chemotherapy, while the other group did not fast. The group that did fast had less negative side effects of chemotherapy. This suggests that the activation of autophagy in their cells helped them clear out the toxins that chemotherapy introduced.

Autophagy is becoming a popular form of treatment for people battling cancer in general. There are a number of blogs you can find of people going through chemotherapy who fast for as long as seven days at a time. They write about losing less hair and having less trouble breathing than most people who go through chemotherapy.

This makes sense because autophagy is getting rid of the leftover toxins from chemotherapy that would otherwise give them harsher side effects. A study of women who had breast cancer showed that women who fasted for over 13 hours a day had lower rates of cancer recurrence. It is truly remarkable how much of a difference it can make.

We can use autophagy to our advantage. Even though we are still waiting to see the pharmaceutical potential of autophagy research, we can stop cancer cells from growing in the first place. Nutrient-rich foods and polyphenol-rich supplements will boost autophagy during our fasts.

Autophagy fights disease in two ways. For one, macroautophagy and chaperone-mediated autophagy directly capture foreign invaders and breaks them down in the lysosome. They prevent bacteria and diseases from within the cell. They prevent the buildup of discarded particles inside the cell and breaks them down for use.

Autophagy also prevents necrosis or the premature death of a cell due to disease or injury. Necrosis creates more cellular garbage that autophagy has to clean up. If you keep cells healthy now by inducing autophagy, they will be less likely to require necrosis, and your autophagy will have less work to do later.

The other way autophagy fights disease is by keeping cells healthy. When cells are healthy, they are better able to fight off disease. Healthy cells make for a healthier immune system, allowing your body to fight off infections more effectively. Healthy cells are better able to keep cancer cells from growing, and if they become cancer cells, they are likely to go through programmed cell death (apoptosis) to save the rest of the body.

The reason we age and eventually die is that our cells lose the ability to perform their functions. They accumulate damage over time and become less effective at their jobs because of it. Autophagy fights against this age-related degradation, so it will help make your cells young again.

Cells age faster when they are not maintained, which makes autophagy the key to anti-aging. Autophagy is your cells' natural way of maintaining themselves; if you never put your cells under stress through starvation or fasting, they will not maintain themselves to a significant degree.

The build-up of proteins due to failed autophagy can lead to Parkinson's disease. This happens because of the degraded membrane leaking.

Alzheimer's disease can develop when the lysosome fails to bond with the autophagosome. This is because the brain cells die when they cannot renew themselves with autophagy, causing the brain to shrink.

A study on mice showed that skeletal muscle fibers showed signs of degeneration because of a lack of autophagy. This led to damaged mitochondria and excessive cell death. It is very good for your body when autophagy removes damaged and dysfunctional mitochondria. Bad mitochondria will release harmful chemicals in your cells. If you increase autophagy, you will reduce the toxic mitochondria in your body.

Much research has been done on the effects of fasting-induced autophagy on skeletal muscles. This part of the body has shown the most significant improvement in autophagy after 36 hours of fasting. If you want to preserve the health of your bones as you age, autophagy is an excellent way to go about it.

A study at the University of Southern California found that fasting for three days has a significant improvement in a person's health. This study was done over six months. Both mice and humans going through chemotherapy participated. The scientists found that white blood cells and other toxins were cleaned out of their systems during the fast. (Normally, white blood cells are good, but since these were people going through chemotherapy, their white blood cells were dead and simply becoming toxic.)

Long-term inflammation and damaged DNA in your cells lead to diseases such as cancer, which means that healthier cells will stave off these problems. Studies show that laboratory mice who underwent less autophagy were more likely to develop cancer.

Autophagy will also improve your digestive health. The cells that make up your gastrointestinal tract are always working. When you activate autophagy, your digestive cells are able to repair themselves, clear themselves of junk, and halt or activate the immune system as needed. In this way, autophagy helps your immune system work more efficiently. Being able to repair this part of your body is critical to the health of your gut.

Until more research comes around that potentially finds a cure for cancer using our new understanding of autophagy, we can use this knowledge to unlock the full potential of autophagy on our bodies and keep them healthy. Any part of your body that is inflamed may be repaired by inducing autophagy.

Since autophagy has been shown to be instrumental in fighting infectious disease, stimulating it is an excellent way to boost your immune system, prevent cancer, and stop other diseases and conditions before they can begin.

Autophagy is better prepared to fight off diseases if you activate it more. The main reason for this is the reduced inflammation autophagy will bring you. The chief way autophagy reduces inflammation is by maintaining homeostasis.

If you have had a poor diet, got little exercise, or smoked, this increased inflammation in your body. Inflammation leads to many diseases and conditions, so reducing it through autophagy is another merit of inducing autophagy.

Both chronic inflammation and excess necrosis can lead to cancer and other diseases. As a whole, your body is better able to do its job when there is less inflammation. Likewise, once you've been fasting and following our autophagy-induced methods for a few months, your altogether healthier body will be able to get even greater health benefit from autophagy.

A healthier body is better able to keep itself healthy and fight disease. If you stay on the course of letting your body naturally detoxify itself, you will feel renewed and even better, live healthier and longer.

This is why we put so much emphasis on consistency. In the beginning, getting into a habit of activating autophagy regularly is more important than fasting for as long as possible.

Don't set high goals for fasting or exercise in the beginning: set goals you know you can achieve, and make it a part of your normal routine. Write down your goals. Once you are able to follow your plan for a few weeks, make your goal harder. Go from a 12-hour fast to a 16-hour fast. We'll talk more about how to make autophagy-based lifestyle goals and how to follow them later on.

Autophagy is always happening in your body in different cells; it just depends on how potent it is. Maintenance mode refers to your cells going through autophagy as normal. Some cells in your body don't have access to food, so they eat their unused proteins and organelles for energy. Maintenance mode will happen whether you fast, exercise, or get enough sleep.

This book is about going beyond the maintenance mode of autophagy. You want to kick autophagy into high gear, so you clear out as many toxins as possible and keep your body at optimal health. Through starvation or fasting, you are able to stimulate autophagy at this potency. Diet and exercise will bring your cells beyond maintenance mode, but not nearly as much as fasting because it puts significantly more stress on your cells.

Beyond the maintenance mode of autophagy is advanced autophagy. Advanced autophagy improves the function of all your cells. Cells free of debris and clutter help the mitochondria work more efficiently.

Chapter 6: Choose the Right Fast for You

There is more than one way to fast, so choose the one that best fits your lifestyle and habits. The most popular is called intermittent fasting.

In this fast, you eat every day, but you also fast for a certain number of hours every day. You can start with a shorter-lasting fast and build up to a longer one.

When you water fast, you consume nothing but water for a period of time. You can do this for 24 hours, or you can go longer to increase the benefits on your body.

There are also other fasts we will cover, such as the 24-hour fast, consecutive-day fasting, and fast mimicking. I'll tell you which ones are best backed up by the research and how to decide which one to follow.

All of them follow the same principle: maximize your autophagy activation by going as long as you can, but not so long that you get sick. Fasting should not make you sick, and if it does, either you are fasting too long, or you are not eating the right foods on your feasting days.

When you water fast, you need to actually consume nothing but water. Water fasts do not allow for juices, coffee, or any other drinks containing nutrients that your body would have to process. Some autophagy enthusiasts spread misinformation that light nutrients from these drinks won't make a difference, but they do. The effects of autophagy from absolute fasting are proved; the effects of autophagy from consuming even small amounts of nutrients are not. Don't negate the whole purpose of autophagy by trying to cheat with beverages.

You can't get away with consuming artificial sweeteners while you fast, either. Even with artificial sweeteners, the vagus nerve is activated because of the smell of food that artificial sweeteners give off. The parasympathetic activation of this nerve causes you to activate mTOR; when you are fasting, you need to give this enzyme the cold shoulder, not even stimulating it with the smell of food. This is true even with things like artificial sweeteners that have no calories.

The same principle applies to other foods as well. Sniffing your pantry probably isn't a great way to stay true to your fast anyway, but it's important to keep in mind that doing so would also stimulate mTOR, therefore slowing autophagy.

People also make the mistake of taking their autophagy-boosting supplements while in their fasting state. You need to save these for your days off of fasting. People do this because they think they don't have enough nutrients to stop autophagy, but this is untrue. Most of these supplements will stop autophagy. Even if some of them don't, you should stay on the safe side and wait until your feasting days.

Many people wonder how long it takes to see the effects of autophagy after they start fasting. One very encouraging fact is that the autophagy of brain cells increases after a pretty short period of fasting of 12 hours. That means even when you simply get a good night of sleep after a day of eating healthful foods, your brain will see a fair amount of autophagy's detox.

Dry fasting is a term that gets thrown around in relation to autophagy, and it is unfortunate. This is a fast where you consume nothing, not even water. We wholeheartedly urge against this. It is very important that you drink water every day. Besides, if one of the perks of autophagy you are seeking is skin health, going without water will totally work against that. Going without any water for even one day can have serious consequences, so do not try the dry fast.

Another strange term that has made its way into the conversation about autophagy is protein fasting. Protein fasting is when you eat nothing but protein, which will not work in your favor for autophagy. You want to consume a moderately low level of protein so that your body burns fat. Fat burns before protein, so consuming less protein helps keep your autophagy as efficient as possible.

It is understandable that you would want to start with intermittent fasting, to begin with. That might be all that you want to do to activate autophagy. However, we do advise you to work yourself up to water fasts.

One of the first effects of water fasting is just what you expect: weight loss. When you don't eat anything, the weight falls off your body pretty fast. Even in just 24 hours, you will go through all the glucagon in your liver.

Once you run out of glucagon, your body starts to run on either protein or fat. In the first few days of a water fast, you will lose about a pound a day. All that said, to be safe. There is no reason for most people to water fast as long as 48 hours, so you are probably fine with a goal of 24 or 36 hours.

The first day of a water fast is always extremely hard, but after you pass this part in the beginning, you start to lose a lot of your cravings. The loss of cravings is one of the perks you get from sticking with a water fast. Cravings make you feel hungry when you do not actually need food, so losing these cravings will help you lose weight and therefore help you be healthier in the long term.

You need to be careful with long-term water fasts. What happens for some people is they are satisfied with the weight they lose during the fast, and then they just go back to their normal diet and sedentary lifestyle. They don't even make fasting a regular part of their lives.

If you want to see results from water fasting, you have to do it consistently. Ideally, you do it a couple of times a week, or even more, if you have a specific reason to make autophagy reach its full potential.

Remember that how much you eat is important, but it is less important than what kinds of food you eat. Foods are meant to provide us with nutrients; when we aren't eating nutrient-rich foods, you aren't going to gain any real health benefit from fasting.

Fasting to activate autophagy is a completely different thing from fasting to "get skinnier." Our goal is not a weight, but improved long-term health.

You should also be aware of something else about long-term water fasting. It comes from the root of the detox that happens from autophagy.

When you induce autophagy by water fasting, all the toxins that were stored in your fat are being released in your body. Since these were stored in your body for so long, losing them all at once can be a very uncomfortable experience.

You may also feel uncomfortable when you lose weight quickly, making your skin feel strange. It can even make you feel sick. But as long as you stay within your limits and are aware that these are just the side effects of water fasting, you will be fine.

The biggest danger of water fasting is veering into the territory of disordered eating. If you fear liking the feeling of fasting too much — if it gives you the kind of feeling that someone might chase with a drug — this is a dangerous road to go down. People who chase a fasting high will continue to fast for continuously longer and longer periods of time to get increased highs.

You want to make sure you are doing it for the right reasons. If you do it to better your health, you will be able to stop if you start feeling legitimately sick.

Even for a water fast, you still need to make sure you have a supply of electrolytes that may not already be in your water at home. Electrolytes are sodium, potassium, calcium, phosphate, and magnesium. You need electrolytes every day to stay healthy, so you still need them on your days water fasting. You can get electrolytes from supplements, you can buy water with electrolytes, or you can make it at home. It just takes water, lemon, and a pinch of salt.

If you are deciding between which fast to do, it depends on what your goals are. If your goals are very ambitious, you might want to go the extra mile and try a long-term water fast. But if you are generally healthy and just want to be as healthy as you can be, intermittent fasting or consecutive day fasting might be closer to what you are looking for.

At the same time, you don't have to limit yourself to one fast or the other. It might be a good idea to make intermittent fasting a part of your regular routine — simply making the window of time during which you eat every day smaller. You can do an intermittent fast on your feasting days and do a full-day fast every other day. If you do this, you are combining intermittent fasting with consecutive day fasting. At the same time, you can choose to spend one day a month to do a 24-hour, 48-hour, or 72-hour water fast. There is more than one way to fast, so you can tailor your fast to what suits your needs and preferences.

One reason you might choose a certain fast over another is for social reasons. It might be hard to convince your friends and family that you are fasting to stimulate autophagy and not just starving yourself. Of course, after reading this book, you will be very knowledgeable about autophagy, so you can explain it to them, but you might not feel like explaining yourself to people all the time. From the social side of things, it might be easier to do intermittent fasting.

We really recommend that you do a 24-hour water fast at least once. People who do it say they have a completely different outlook on their eating habits after they do it. The water fast makes people realize how accustomed they are to putting food in their mouth throughout the day; there is no better way to confront the cravings that we usually succumb to.

When your fast is over, you have to make sure to break the fast the right way. If you introduce carbohydrate-rich foods into your body right after a fast, your body is forced to introduce a rush of insulin in order to digest these carbs. The rush of insulin will require a lot of phosphate, potassium, magnesium, and vitamins. Since you just went through a fast, your body might not have all of these vitamins available. If you fed yourself the carbs anyway, this could lead to heart failure, hypertension, and even death in the most extreme cases.

When you break a fast, be sure not to consume a significant amount of carbs. Whatever your first meal after a fast is, it needs to be low in carbs if it has carbs at all.

There are specific steps you need to take when breaking a fast. You have to supplement yourself with thymine and other B vitamins thirty minutes before you start eating.

You also need to start slow. You can't introduce a lot of solid foods into your body right away. The first meal after a fast should be 10 calories per kilogram of your body weight. Drink water and also make sure you have electrolytes just like when you were fasting.

You should also drink some juice, but it shouldn't be a brand with a ton of sugar and preservatives.

At this stage of breaking the fast, it's better to eat in many small snacks as opposed to in a few large meals. Slowly introduce small portions to your body.

There is one consistent trend in human studies about fasting, and it is a trend that you could look at positively or negatively. In pretty much every study where humans were asked to fast, there was a high drop-out rate for fasting. They either dropped out near the beginning, or they fasted for a while, but then didn't keep up with it.

This trend shouldn't make you think it's impossible to stick with fasting. After all, there were still participants who stuck with fasting. But it is a clear sign that fasting is hard to do and hard to keep doing.

Based on all the research currently available in this rapidly growing area of knowledge, we recommend doing two kinds of fasts simultaneously.

The first one is intermittent fasting. Follow the keto diet on your off-days and follow a decent fast on your on-days. A decent fast can even be eating breakfast in the morning and then not eating until the next day. Once you get used to it, this will just start to feel normal.

The second kind of fast doesn't replace the intermittent fast, but it goes with it. As well as doing a shorter but decently long fast every other day, fast for longer one day every month. Unless you are really looking to go above and beyond, a fast of 24 hours will be sufficient for this longer fasting day. More important than the length of this fast is how many times a month you can do it. For most people, twice a month should give you all the detox you need.

Chapter 7: Diet and Supplements

To begin with, we want to issue a warning. You should avoid supplements and medications that claim to induce autophagy. As of today, no supplements that make such claims are real. Biologists are still working on such a drug, but we are not there yet.

People are always looking for the easy way of doing things. The hard way is simple, if not easy: fasting, diet, exercise, and plenty of deep sleep. Anyone who thinks they can activate autophagy with a medicine without doing these things is wrong, at least at this point.

If you are doing a water fast and you eat anything at all, you lose all of the benefits of stimulating autophagy. Even consuming 50 calories makes your insulin go back up dramatically, turning off autophagy — so be sure not to eat at all during these periods.

It will be hard at first, but you are capable of enduring the initial discomfort so you can get the health benefits. To stay healthy, you should activate autophagy in every organ in your body, including your lungs and your heart. But one of the most active organs in activating autophagy is the liver.

When we talk about supplements, you need to understand that supplements need to go together with a diet or rich, natural foods. Supplements won't help you in the long run if you are not also eating healthy.

Omega-3 fats are a healthy kind of fat that everyone should include in their diet. They are vital to the elasticity of your cells, which is a great benefit for the health of your cells for autophagy. It is common for people to take supplements to get omega-3 fats, but we actually advise against doing this. There is scientific evidence that omega-3 fats positive affect health outcomes when they are consumed via foods in one's diet, and there is no evidence that getting omega-3 fats from supplements will give you this same benefit.

The same idea goes for all the supplements we talk about. If you aren't going to get these nutrients from your normal diet, getting them through supplements is probably going to be better than not getting them at all. But it's far better if you get them from the foods you eat.

Sadly, since factory farms are the source of meat for most grocery stores, omega-3 fats are hard to come by in modern grocery stores. The animals that provide this meat do not live in a natural environment. Instead of grazing on the grass that would indirectly give you nutrients from eating their meat, these animals are fed numerous chemicals and are given steroids to increase their bulk.

It is true that you can improve a lot of markers of health with caloric restriction, but it isn't as effective as intermittent fasting. Reducing your caloric intake by 10% can improve blood sugar, blood pressure, and cholesterol, but it is less backed by data than fasting-induced autophagy.

You do have many choices for how you want to fast. You can do a 24-hour fast, a consecutive day fast, intermittent fasting, and water fasting. When you water fast, you consume nothing but water.

If you don't like vegetables, you should consider putting them in a blender and mixing them with some fruits. (But don't add too much fruit, because they are high in glucose, so they severely affect your blood sugar.)

Green tea increase AMPK, the enzyme that increases autophagy. Green tea works extremely well in tandem with tumeric, which more directly activates autophagy. Basically, green tea increases the potential of autophagy, while tumeric pretty much activates it. This is not to say that you can forget about fasting and exercise, relying on tumeric alone. But if you activate autophagy with these practices and enjoy green tea and tumeric, autophagy will be even more effective.

The reishi mushroom is another thing you should consider adding to your diet. It reduces the growth of colon cancer cells by suppressing the phosphorylation of the P38 protein. Essentially, the P38 protein would normally help colon cancer cells grow by suppressing autophagy in non-cancerous cells, and the chemicals in the reishi mushroom prevent this from happening.

What is great about autophagy-boosting foods is that they allow you to approach autophagy from many angles. If you incorporate them into your diet, you will activate autophagy through fasting, increase its potency with green tea, and suppresses the blocking of autophagy with reishi mushrooms, just as one example.

One way to look at boosting autophagy is as fun. You can approach the maximization of autophagy from several different angles. If you cover as many bases as you can, you will unlock the greatest possible potential for autophagy. There are always new things we are learning about autophagy — even though this book gives you a very thorough rundown of what we know at this point, it doesn't hurt to do your own research every month or so to see what autophagy enthusiasts and scientists have discovered recently.

This book has examined all the opinions of health experts and methods so far and came to a conclusion on the best ways to activate autophagy, and with all the knowledge it will give you, you will be able to do your own research with a very informed perspective. You won't be misled by false information or unhealthy diet tips.

On your feasting days, there are several foods you should eat to get the most out of your water fasting. There are supplements available, too.

These days, you can find all kinds of information about the keto diet and what foods it includes, but the basic principle is always the same: you want to consume more healthy fats than carbohydrates.

The goal of a keto diet is to make your body go into ketosis. Ketosis is when you release a great influx of ketones, which are fat-burning molecules. Your body enters ketosis when you don't give it carbohydrates to burn — it tends to favor burning carbs for energy before other chemicals, leaving you with extra fat if you have a diet high in carbs.

The role of insulin is to increase the storage of energy, but it also creates a lot of fat. Getting to a low level of insulin is not all that counts, but staying at a low level of insulin for a long period of time. This is what will really stimulate autophagy, and the Keto diet will help you get there.

By following the keto diet, not only will your body burn more fat because you have fewer carbs for it to burn first, but you will have a surge in the number of ketones available to burn fat.

The keto diet and an autophagy-stimulating lifestyle do not necessarily have to go together. Either of them will make you healthier and boost autophagy on their own. Since carbs take so long to burn, eating a lot of them makes the start of autophagy after fasting much later. A healthy diet will help you digest your food and activate autophagy within 4 hours; if you eat a meal with many carbs and then stop eating, it will take about 8 hours to start autophagy.

What makes the keto diet so effective is it forces your cells to use autophagy to consume your good fats and their own damaged organelles along with other cytoplasm instead of constantly staying busy with breaking down carbohydrates. When you eat a lot of carbs, your cells are too busy breaking those down to break down the cellular garbage in your body.

Let's talk about the different stages your body goes into when you are fasting and following the keto diet on your feasting days.

After 12 hours, you enter the metabolic state called ketosis. Your body starts to break down and burn its fat. Some of the fat goes to the liver to make ketone bodies or ketones. Ketones are an alternative to glucose for a source of energy for your cells.

The fact that your brain cells use ketones when you are fasting is the reason why people report feeling clearer in the head when they fast.

Ketosis will also help improve your mood. Ketones produce fewer inflammatory products than glucose, as well.

After 18 hours of fasting, you switch to fat-burning mode. Now, you are making even more ketones. Your level of ketones is now significantly higher than it would normally be.

Within 24 hours, your cells are doing a great job of recycling old components from their cellular waste.

By 48 hours, you are reaching your peak of potential from ketosis. The increase of ketones increases your growth hormones. Growth hormones are good to have because they produce lean muscle mass and reduce the accumulation of fat tissue, which is especially great as we age.

There is even research connecting growth hormones to higher longevity in mammals, as well as cardiovascular health and wound healing.

Within 54 hours of ketosis, the level of insulin in your body is at the lowest it has been so far. Your body is also more sensitive to insulin compared to before.

Lowering your insulin has many benefits, both in the short term and in the long term. Lowered insulin puts a stopper on the signaling pathways that mTOR uses, which would otherwise suppress autophagy. Lowered insulin also reduces inflammation.

After 72 hours of ketosis, your body is breaking down old immune cells and making new ones.

While the keto diet elegantly complements an autophagy-activating lifestyle, ketosis is not required to undergo autophagy.

Because of this, you will want to eat a low-carb diet even if you don't follow the keto diet. That said, we recommend that you at least try the keto diet so you can see the difference for yourself.

Much like autophagy, the first thing people tend to notice is the weight loss — but they go far beyond losing weight. It might seem like too much to start fasting and change your diet at the same time, so you should try to get used to one and decide if you want to try the other.

People tend to underestimate the importance of the nutrients in the foods they eat when they aren't fasting. Since you aren't eating when you're fasting, this makes the healthiness of the foods you consume on your non-fasting days even more important.

Sometimes people can get intimidated by all the information about nutrition that they hear. But it is a lot simpler than people think. What they are missing is this simple rule in nutrition: pay attention to the number of calories in your food compared to how many nutrients it has.

If your food is high in calories but low in nutrients, you shouldn't be eating it on your feasting days. These are foods like waffles covered in chocolate and strawberries; they are certainly high in calories, but they do no favors for your health.

You have to choose foods like vegetables, protein-rich meats with good fats, and some fruit.

In general, you want to avoid consuming a lot of calories. Every calorie you put into your body takes time for your body to digest, which will greatly diminish the amount of time that you are actually fasting.

This is not to add fuel to the misleading idea that calories are bad. Calories themselves are neutral — it is the nutrients your calories contain that matter.

There are even more autophagy-boosting foods you should consider adding to your diet: cayenne pepper, medicinal mushrooms, apple cider vinegar, blueberries, and cruciferous vegetables such as broccoli.

Just remember that foods that are not directly autophagy-boosting should still be part of your diet, as long as they do not contain high levels of nutrients that suppress autophagy, such as carbs. A healthy diet includes a wide variety of foods. This remains true when you make fasting-induced autophagy a part of your regular routine.

Be sure you aren't depriving yourself of Vitamin D. This vitamin is necessary for many of the processes in your body, including autophagy. If you don't have enough of it, it will seriously hinder your detox. Doing this is easy enough — just be sure to get some sun exposure every day. If you are careful and use sunblock, you can get the benefits of sunlight without harming your skin. If you can't get direct sun exposure every day, take a vitamin D supplement.

These foods do not put you into autophagy alone; there is no special food or drug that will do all that work for you. The only way to enjoy the full benefits of autophagy is following the tips we give you, but mostly the fundamentals that we keep reminding you of: good sleep, regular exercise, a keto diet (or at least a diet low in carbs and high in nutrients), and fasting.

But even though these foods don't start up autophagy on their own, but they do boost it by depleting your energy levels. They deplete energy from your cells, making it more likely that your fast will induce their stress response, and they will eat their cellular junk for food. As an added benefit, these foods are especially good for your brain cells.

~

People who are in ketosis are able to go through significant autophagy every night when they go to sleep. This is because they have a lot of good fats in their systems.

Let's get into what ketosis really is. It's a metabolic process that happens when your body begins to burn fat for energy because it doesn't have many carbohydrates.

When this happens, the liver produces chemicals called ketones. The keto diet aims to induce ketosis so you can burn more fat. It is obvious why this has become so popular recently, because who doesn't want to burn the fat on their body?

If you mix a keto diet with autophagy, you won't be keeping that loose skin either, because autophagy will increase the amount of collagen available to your skin cells, keeping your skin tighter and more youthful.

The strange thing about calling the ketogenic diet a diet is that it really includes all the foods you should be eating to live healthily and take care of your body. It is not so much a diet as it is what you should be eating to stay healthy.

This is not to say there are not ways of following the keto diet that are unhealthy. Even though the fats of the keto diet are good fats, it is still possible to overindulge in them and harm your gut.

We have talked about all the reasons you should fast, but at the end of the day, it is your choice how you want to activate autophagy. One alternative method you can consider fasting is simply following the keto diet. If you allow plenty of time between your ketogenic meals, you are still intermittent fasting, so you will still get some of the health benefits of autophagy from doing this. A keto diet alone won't optimize autophagy by any means, but it is still another option for you to choose from.

When we say you should reduce the protein you consume on your feasting days, we should get more specific about what we mean. On feasting days, you should limit your protein to about 20 grams.

A lot of Americans have diets where over half of the nutrients they consume are carbohydrates. The keto diet turns this typical diet upside down. In a keto diet, you don't eat more than 25 grams of carbs a day. It does an amazing job of complementing autophagy because autophagy loves good fats and hates cholesterol.

The feeling of hunger is most closely attributed to your blood sugar level. The higher it is, the less hungry you will feel. The lower it is, the less hungry you will feel. The best way to make your blood sugar feel high is limiting the carbohydrates in your diet. When you eat a lot of carbs, you are forcing your body to process a lot of nutrients that don't actually increase your blood sugar.

A chemical found in grapes called resveratrol can stimulate AMPK, and therefore induce autophagy.

When you put yourself on a keto diet, what you are really trying to do is put yourself in ketosis so you will burn fat cells.

Fat is an important source of energy that can absorb vitamins and minerals. We need it to create cell membranes, and the sheathes that surround nerves. We also need fat for muscle movement, blood clotting, and reducing inflammation.

But when it comes to your long-term health, some fats are better than others. Good fats include polyunsaturated fats and monounsaturated fats. The absolutely bad fats are trans fats that do not naturally occur and are now banned in the United States.

Saturated fats are somewhere between good and bad. Good fats mostly come from vegetables, nuts, seeds, and fish. Doctors recommend that you get about 30 percent of your calories from good fats.

It turns out that fat is not the one thing that is causing the obesity epidemic. Gaining weight is mostly the result of consuming a lot of calories and then not burning them.

You mostly get omega-3 fats from fatty fish such as trout, salmon, mackerel, and catfish. You can also get it from flaxseed and walnuts. The American Heart Association recommends that we eat two servings of fatty fish every week.

Trans fats are prominent in the foods in the typical American diet, such as baked goods, fried foods, icing, crackers, cookies, packaged snacks, margarine, and microwave popcorn. The U.S. Dietary Guidelines recommends that you keep your trans fat intake to less than 2 grams per day. Trans fats have no nutritional value to speak of. But eliminating trans fats from your diet is not enough to be healthy. You need to keep up an exercise regimen and eat other nutritional foods while you eat healthy fats.

Monounsaturated and polyunsaturated fats are essential for unclogging your arteries, so you need to make sure they get into your diet.

Saturated fats are in the middle because you want to keep them to about 10% of your total calories every day, or less if possible. Saturated fats and trans fats raise your cholesterol, clog your arteries, and increase your risk for heart disease when they make up too many of your calories.

People in Mediterranean countries tend to consume a lot of unsaturated fat in the form of olive oil. Their low levels of heart disease are usually credited to these unsaturated fats.

Polyunsaturated fats are mostly found in vegetable oils, and they help lower your blood cholesterol levels. Where you can substitute saturated fats with polyunsaturated fats, substitute them. Omega-3 fats are a type of polyunsaturated fat.

Remember that reducing your fat intake does not reduce your risk of cancer directly. But it will make you lose weight, which itself will decrease your risk of cancer.

The risk of cancer is something that the demographic of overweight menopausal women, in particular, should be aware of. If you belong to this group, you should follow the guidance in this book to help you lose weight and greatly lower this risk.

Polyunsaturated fats are particularly important because they are essential to your body, and your body can't make them on their own.

Saturated fat is bad for you because it drives up total cholesterol. It causes blockages to form at the arteries leading to the heart and other parts of your body.

The chemical structure of fats is a chain of carbon atoms bonded to hydrogen atoms. Healthier unsaturated fats are bonded to fewer hydrogens, while unhealthy saturated fats are bonded to more hydrogens.

We'll close the chapter by talking about some of the foods you should introduce to your diet that will help activate autophagy or boost its effects.

Green tea is the easiest thing you can consume that will boost autophagy. The active ingredient of green tea that does this is EGCG. This chemical targets autophagy, specifically in the liver. The health of your liver is crucial to your overall health, so enjoying a cup or two of green tea every day is only going to improve your health.

Ginger is another autophagy-boosting food. It contains a chemical called 6-shogaol that prevents the cells in your lungs from growing too rapidly, which is a great benefit if you are trying to prevent lung cancer. It will regulate the process of autophagy so your cells can clean out cancer-causing agents that are already present in your lungs.

Caffeine lowers your risk of degenerative diseases, which is one of our goals in activating autophagy.

Olive oil will also help induce autophagy, but be wary of the brand you get. Many olive oil brands are not authentic — make sure you get the real deal.

CBD oil is one of the active cannabinoids found in the cannabis plant. Unlike the other active cannabinoid, THC, CBD is not psychoactive, so it does not make you high. But it can be used to help treat many diseases by reducing inflammation. Research has found that CBD enhances autophagy pathways in the brain.

Scientists say that over half of people are at risk of deficient Vitamin D. All of the tissues in your body have receptors for Vitamin D. If you don't get enough of it, it can lead to serious physical and psychological consequences. Vitamin D can be found in many foods, or you can get it from the sunlight.

Chapter 8: Helpful Facts about Autophagy

This chapter is all about giving you all of the information you might possibly need about autophagy and how to increase it in your body. These facts should be both helpful and interesting, so take a look through them and see if you can find something that will help you.

The Glucose-Ketone Index

You should also know a quantitative measure that can tell you if you are going through autophagy. No method is completely accurate, but this one is the best one you can get, and you can do it at home with a blood sugar meter. You will have to prick your finger to do this, which you may not want to do — but if you really want to get the most accurate possible idea of your level of autophagy, this is how you will do it. We have discussed the qualitative ways to tell if you are going through autophagy, but it is also worthwhile to discuss the quantitative ones.

For starters, to get a good measurement of your autophagy using the glucose-ketone index, you have to be fasting at the moment that you use to take the blood sugar test. This might seem obvious, but just be sure you are at least 12 hours into a fast when you take the test. Otherwise, you won't get an accurate result. If you aren't fasting, your body has glucose in it right now, so the test won't measure your autophagy at all.

This quantitative measure of autophagy uses the glucose-ketone index formula. A blood sugar meter will tell you your level of glucose and your level of blood ketones. The formula goes like this: you take your blood glucose, and you divide it by your blood ketones; before you divide by ketones, you divide the glucose by 18. (But only divide glucose by 18 if your device measures your glucose in mmol/L. If it already measures glucose in mg/dL, you can leave the number as it is.) You take the glucose/ketones number and divide it by 3.4. This will tell you your glucose-ketone index.

Let's go talk about what this number means.

If your index is below 3, that means you are a very high level of ketosis. You don't want your number to get this low. This index value can be an indicator of epilepsy or cancer.

If your index is between 3 and 6, this is a sign of obesity, type-2 diabetes, or insulin resistance. You don't want this value as your index, either.

An index between 6 and 9 is a sign of optimal health. If your index is between these numbers, you are in a good position to lose or maintain weight. When you go through autophagy, you want to go for an index between 6 and 9. If you go above 9, there is no ketosis, and you are not going through significant autophagy.

Remember that even though this is the most quantitative measure you can get, it isn't absolutely accurate.

If you go a little below 6, this isn't a definitive indicator that you are on the verge of weight gain. Similarly, if you are between 6 and 9, this isn't the ultimate indicator of health. You should use other signs of health and continue going to your doctor. Listen to what they have to say about the state of your health; don't rely on the ketone-glucose index alone. It is just one fairly accurate way to measure the extent of your autophagy.

The reason this index isn't always totally reliable is that your blood sugar levels are influenced by many different factors, and it's nearly impossible to nail down whether they go down because of autophagy. If you are somewhere between 3 and 9 on the index, you are probably fine. This measurement is best used along with qualitative measures such as weight loss, skin health, and simply how you feel. The last one might seem unscientific, but you should feel significantly healthier after balancing your autophagy with a healthy lifestyle for an extended period. That feeling will be incredibly satisfying, so as you keep track of your autophagy in other ways, don't lose sight of your newfound happiness.

When You Should Eat

Don't only focus on how much you eat, but also the times that you eat.

Your body is better able to process food at earlier times in the day. When you are getting started fasting and changing your diet, you should begin with getting your most important nutrients early in the day, and then eat less later in the day.

Try the Water Fast

We highly recommend that you try to do one long water fast where you set your goal decently high, just so you can see what you are capable of. If you think you can healthily stand it, try to aim for a 24-hour water fast first. This means consuming no calories for 24 hours.

After you fast for 24 hours, you'll realize how much cleaner your body feels. You will also have a clearer mind.

Common Mistakes

There are a lot of common mistakes people make when stimulating autophagy, so let's go over them so you can be prepared and try to avoid them.

One is not fasting long enough. If you only fast for 16 hours, you are really only fasting for 12 hours since it takes your body 4 hours to digest your last meal. When you are still digesting food, you are not going through autophagy, because there is still food in your body. Your cells are experiencing none of the stress that is required to start up autophagy.

If you stop eating at Noon and don't eat again until Midnight, you only fasted for 8 hours. Autophagy will occur more than it does over this time period than it will when there are only a few hours between meals, but this level of autophagy is dwarfed in comparison to the detox you will get from a true 16-hour fast.

Another common mistake is drinking coffee. Coffee has fats in it that your cells will eat for nutrients; if your body is processing the fats from coffee, you are not going through any significant autophagy.

Another common mistake is underestimating the importance of a good night of sleep. It's better to go to bed earlier after a day of fasting; most of your autophagy will happen when you are in a deep sleep, and going to bed early will help you spend more of your time resting in a deep sleep. You may think sleep is secondary when it comes to autophagy, but it is the glue of autophagy activation that makes all the positive effects possible. Be sure to prioritize these early hours of sleep to get the most out of the autophagy from your fast.

Most of autophagy happens when you are asleep, so it is better to go to bed on an empty stomach. This is yet another way to get the most out of natural detox your cells will perform while you are unconscious.

Your brain's melatonin is necessary to activate autophagy in your neurons. We will say it once again: it really matters that you get enough sleep. In today's world, part of sleeping well at night is avoiding blue lights. It might seem impossible, but if you try to stay away from screens once it gets dark out, you will notice a considerable improvement in your sleep. You can even wear glasses that block out blue lights and adjust the display settings on your devices to lower white and blue lights.

Consistency

I know we beat the dead horse with this point, but it matters a lot: consistency is critical to the effectiveness of autophagy. Maybe the most common mistake people make when stimulating autophagy is not doing it often enough. They think doing one long fast a year will be sufficient, but this is wrong.

It is better for you to do one shorter fast every month than one 48-hour fast a year. Detoxifying the body is a long-term project. You can't expect to get it all done once a year and be done.

You don't want to be a perfectionist about autophagy. If you fall out of your habits for a few months, you can always start again. The next time, start slower.

Make your first goal really easy. Don't let yourself eat after dinner — let's say, don't let yourself eat after 7pm. If you make it until 7am the next day without eating, you have already done a 12-hour fast. It might not seem like a lot, but it helps you realize that fasting longer is simply tacking more hours onto these 12 hours.

At this point, you continue increasing the duration of your fasts by a couple hours at a time. Go from 12 to 15, to 18, and so on.

It doesn't matter what time you choose to fast, either. You can skip breakfast and lunch and save your meal for dinner. You can eat only in the morning. In this book, we recommend intermittent fasting, where you fast for some period every other day and eat normally on the other days. This is because it helps you remember the importance of balancing introducing nutrients to your body to stimulate cell growth on the feasting days and the importance of detoxifying your cells through autophagy on your fasting days.

Some sources claim that fasting for longer than 12 hours is unnecessary, but this doesn't bear out in the research. The most relevant study showed that people who fasted for 24 hours had 3 times the number of autophagosomes in their cells; people who fasted for 36 hours had 20% autophagosomes. This suggests that the biggest leap in autophagy happens after about 24 hours of fasting, and 12 hours of fasting isn't going to get you there.

Don't take the fact that autophagy stops increasing as much after 24 hours as meaning there is no reason to fast more than 24 hours. Indeed, 24 hours is an effective length for a fast, and if you stop there, you did well for your body. But if you hang in there for even longer, even if your autophagosomes stop increasing as dramatically, your body will continue to stay in advanced autophagy and detoxify your cells more.

That said, the way you fast depends heavily on your own health profile. This is why it is so important that you talk to your doctor about fasting if you have any health problems. With this in mind, you should strive for longer fasts if possible, because it will allow you to get the most out of autophagy.

You don't want to start with long periods of fasting right away, because your body has to adjust to the pattern of eating. At first, it will be used to you eating several times a day. Immediately trying a 48-hour fast might seem appealing at first, but it is unlikely your body will accept this because it is too new. You will burn yourself out if you don't give yourself time to get used to it.

As your body adapts, it will get used to long periods of time without food. Ultimately, this will be better for your body. Stick with fasting during the uncomfortable periods, and you will feel the results.

Start with simple goals. Start with one realistic goal: you want to fast for 12 hours the next day. All this takes is eating breakfast at 7am and then waiting to eat until dinner at 7pm. You can even make a smaller goal if you would like to. It doesn't matter how intense your fasts are in the beginning; the important thing is getting used to fasting and making it a normal part of your life.

Don't Neglect Exercise

People also think exercise isn't that important when they are fasting. On the contrary, exercise is one of the best ways to trigger autophagy. Whatever your level of physical fitness, you need to incorporate exercise into your fasting days.

We've mostly talked about studies on the effects of fasting on autophagy, but there is also plenty of research on exercise and autophagy. When mice in a lab were put on a training regimen where they did a lot of running, scientists found they had increased numbers of autophagosomes as a result. This led them to believe that training in cardio is a good way to activate autophagy.

Eat Less Protein, Sometimes

Since autophagy recycles the protein that is already in your body, it is good to reduce your protein consumption from time to time. But you still want normal protein levels at other times so your cells can grow healthily.

But keep this in mind: for many people, their idea of "normal" protein consumption is far too high. An easy way to figure out how much protein you should eat is multiplying your weight by 0.8. The result is in grams of protein. Easy!

There is another useful side-note that you should keep in mind. Not only do people tend to think they need more protein than is really healthy for them, but they tend to get their protein from processed meats they buy at the market. We know how expensive and inaccessible grass-fed meats can be to attain, but on the whole, it would be better for your body if you kept these meats out of your system.

The preservation methods used in these meats have been suggested to cause cancer even more than smoking in some studies. These few studies don't prove anything, but the consensus among nutritionists is that you should avoid eating a lot of red meat anyway. You are probably better safe than sorry.

Protein cycling works very well in tandem with fasting. It allows you to spend your feasting days eating nutrient-rich foods that boost autophagy, and your fasting days activating autophagy by putting stress on your cells. The lower-than-usual proportions of protein will make it much easier for your cells to go through their detox.

Protein Cycling

Another strategy to try is called protein cycling. What you do here is changing between periods of low protein consumption and normal protein consumption. You want periods of normal consumption because protein is essential to your body's health, but you also want periods of low protein, so you activate autophagy, and it recycles the protein it already has. You see, if you tend to consume high volumes of protein every day, you are simply adding more waste for your cells to clean up, greatly hindering your efforts in stimulating autophagy. Autophagy will still occur when you fast, but it will be less effective because it is busy recycling all the protein in your diet. Protein cycling prevents this problem by decreasing your overall intake, especially for the days you fast.

The same principles that go for fasting go for protein cycling. You don't want to go through long periods with low protein. If you deprive yourself of protein too much because protein is, in fact, essential to your body's well-being. But you still want to go through periods of low protein, so your body activates autophagy without excess protein to deal with. Since we generally recommend intermittent fasting in this book, we suggest that you consume a normal amount of protein every other feasting day, and low amounts of protein on the other feasting days.

Diversify Your Autophagy-Activating Methods

If you don't activate autophagy, your cells lag behind because of the dead weight of their damaged organelles, discarded proteins, and other proteins that are no longer helping them perform their functions. They will do some amount of autophagy on their own, but without you putting them into stress for long periods, they will be stuck with these half-eaten particles and organelles without putting them to use. These dead weights in your cells become toxic if they linger long enough.

When we talk about detoxifying our bodies through autophagy, we are not only talking about clearing out toxins that enter the cells from the outside, although autophagy will also take care of these. We are also talking about the unused particles that were once parts of your cells. When they stay in your cells' cytoplasm for long enough without playing any role in the cell, they reduce the efficiency of the cell. They are partly the cause of the effects of aging. When this happens in billions of cells across your body, this means your body, in general, is less able to function the right way.

Since your cells form every part of your body, our goal is to improve your health by starting with these microscopic building blocks.

The best way to stimulate autophagy and maximize it when it does happen is to approach it from several different angles.

You need to follow a special autophagy-enhancing diet for your feasting days, follow your fasting days strictly, get at least eight hours of sleep (when most of the autophagy will occur), and exercise regularly to induce stress in your cells.

Even though you need to approach autophagy from all these angles, you still have a lot of choices. Your exercise, diet, and fasting should be fine-tuned to your needs and preferences. This ensures that you will be able to activate autophagy consistently without getting burned out.

If you set your goals too high too early, you will get burned out and quit completely. You have to start slow and increase your goals as you are able.

Let's go over your different options so you can decide what best suits you.

When you start making your plan of attack for activating autophagy, you need to keep something in mind. One lifestyle change will not be enough to activate autophagy. If you fast every other day but eat tons of snack foods and carbohydrates when you aren't fasting, you might as well not fast. You aren't going to induce real autophagy because it takes your body a long time to digest these kinds of foods.

Autophagy doesn't start until your body is done digesting your food. This means that even if you follow the keto diet on your non-fasting days, your fast doesn't truly begin until four hours after you finish eating. When you eat foods that aren't part of the keto diet, it takes even longer.

Fasting itself makes autophagy simple because all you have to do is consume zero calories on your fasting days. But it still requires that you live healthily outside of your fasts.

I'll try not to repeat this too much, but it is important: besides fasting, get eight hours of quality sleep every night and exercise regularly, ideally 20-30 minutes a day. These are really just as simple as fasting, so be sure to do them, and your fasting-induced autophagy will cleanse your body thoroughly. In the next chapter, you'll learn more about the importance of sleep and exercise in autophagy.

The enzyme mTOR is responsible for cell growth. Cell growth is a vital part of our system, but too much growth leads to excessive cellular waste.

When mTOR is inactive, autophagy is active. You need to understand that mTOR is not absolutely bad, and autophagy is not absolutely bad. Ideally, you alternate between days of following an autophagy-boosting diet low in carbohydrates and days of fasting to activate autophagy. During autophagy, your body will remove toxins; when you eat and activate the mTOR enzyme, you grow new cells. This is the perfect balance that you should aim for.

Fasting is the most effective way we know of to induce autophagy. When we fast, our insulin goes down, making the hormone glucagon go up.

Glucagon is what ultimately activates autophagy. It causes us to get nutrients from cleaning out old parts to make new ones. Our bodies' cells have to clear out space for new cells before they have made new ones, and they also new materials from the breakdown of cellular garbage to form new parts.

On the other side of things, what stops autophagy the most is eating. As glucose goes up, your glucagon goes down, making autophagy stop. Even eating a small amount of food stops autophagy completely. This is why certain diets may boost autophagy when it occurs, but they won't activate autophagy on their own.

As I tell you throughout the book, you must find a healthy balance in your cycle between eating nutrient-rich foods and fasting to activate autophagy. If you focus too much on autophagy, the toxins your cells broke down will go without the use and turn back into waste. If you focus too much on diet, you will rarely go through autophagy, and when you do, it will be for short periods of time. If you want to really detoxify your body, you need to put your body in autophagy for a significant period of time.

Alternating between periods of eating healthy foods to build new cells and periods of fasting to clean out your existing cells with autophagy is the key to living a long and healthy life.

You can increase your cellular metabolic rate simply by eating less, which leads to less wear and tear on your cells from the process of metabolism. You need to give your body food to produce new cells, but you can limit how many calories you take in while doing this and decrease the overall damage done to your cells.

The balance between a healthy diet and inducing autophagy does not only mean that you need to balance good food with effective fasting. You should also take note of how these two things complement one another. If you fast consistently and force your cells to break down toxins, they have simpler parts to build organelles from. If you eat healthy on your feasting days, the enzyme mTOR will cause your cells to make something out of these parts through anabolism.

This part of the balance I am sure you understand by now. But let's talk about how mTOR and AMPK complement each other. If your cells make healthier parts through anabolism as a result of mTOR, your healthier cells will be more effective the next time they undergo autophagy. This is a beautiful cycle that should remind you: mTOR is not a bad enzyme, and AMPK is not a good enzyme. When you let both of them perform their roles to their fullest extent, that is what will give you the most health benefit.

By now, you have probably gotten this idea, but I'll say it explicitly: activating autophagy to its fullest extent requires a lot of lifestyle changes. There is no magic bullet that you can get all the same health benefits from. To get every benefit, you have to fast consistently and live a healthy life outside of your fasts.

The Benefits of Autophagy over Caloric Restriction

The research on restricting calories alone is mixed. Some studies suggest that it improves human health and lifespan, and some suggest it does not. Although it is interesting to note that the studies that did not support that caloric restriction increases lifespan, it did support the hypothesis that caloric restriction reduces aging. Both autophagy and caloric restriction focus on the effect of cellular processes on your general health that happens under the surface.

In principle, caloric restriction makes sense. It follows the facts we know about biology. Metabolism slowly degrades your cells, so caloric restriction lessens the damage to your cells. This keeps them living longer. This way,

The good news is you will get the benefits of autophagy without thinking about caloric restriction simply by way of fasting. If caloric restriction indeed increases lifespan and health, you will get these benefits too.

Cardio vs. Resistance Training Exercise

While the autophagy study on mice who did cardio showed increased autophagosomes, we know from other research that strength and resistance training are the best kind of exercise to stimulate autophagy. In fact, building muscle is the best way to activate autophagy through exercise. It is probably the second most effective method, just behind fasting.

Resistance training improves the resistance of your muscle cells, putting them into stress, and giving them a heavier food requirement. They fulfill this requirement by tapping into their stores of excess proteins and dead organelles.

Autophagy protects your muscles and helps to prevent age-related muscle loss. At the same time, having more muscle mass makes you healthier overall, which further improves the effectiveness of your autophagy.

Some studies suggest that even a little bit of resistance training goes further for autophagy than a lot of fasting. Even if this is true, of course, why not get the best of both worlds? Boost autophagy by keeping active and routinely fasting.

Everyone loves that refreshing feeling after they exercise. This feeling comes from autophagy; it is your muscle cells repairing themselves after you make microscopic tears on their tissue during your workout.

The short-term acute stress induced by resistance training such as weight lifting is the best way to induce autophagy. You should aim for this kind of exercise at least 20 to 30 minutes every day if you want to optimize your health.

Getting into a habit of exercise is no different from getting into a habit of eating. You can't be a perfectionist about it. If your initial goal is to exercise twice a week and you don't get around to it, don't give up. Write down the goal again and try it again.

Autophagy Quotes

"Most processed foods and ingredients are low in protein, high in carbs, high in fat, and engineered to increase palatability. They're literally designed by scientists to make you overeat because you're not getting enough protein for satiety, no micronutrients, and way too many over-stimulating sugars and other ingredients that make you lose your sanity." Siim Land, *Metabolic Autophagy: Practice Intermittent Fasting and Resistance Training to Build Muscle and Promote Longevity*

"Fasting is more ancestrally appropriate. It is what we did in a time when humans were generally healthier. We ate when the sun came up and stopped when it went down." -thehartofhealth.com

"Life is an equilibrium state between synthesis and degradation of proteins." -Yoshinori Ohsumi

"I am just a basic cell biologist who has been working with yeast for almost 40 years. I would like to take this opportunity to note my appreciation for the many lessons and wonderful gifts from yeast — perhaps my favorite of all being sake and liquor." - Yoshinori Ohsumi

"Caloric restriction triggers autophagy, a cell-recycling process where your body clears out damaged or dead cells." - thehartofhealth.com

"Intermittent fasting definitely and massively increases autophagy, and thanks to our caveman history, it thrived. In times of little food, lysosomes would race around the body looking for damaged cells, pre-diseased cells, and cells that weren't doing much. It would chop them apart — into their smallest parts — and either burn them for energy or use them to repair other areas. Simply put, it would perform miracles without any outside help." Robert Skinner

"Hands and lips and teeth, and you'd forgotten—no, you'd never known— this way of knowing someone, this dissolution of self, this autophagy." Alaya Dawn Johnson

Chapter 9: How to Be Safe While Maximizing Autophagy

As we have emphasized throughout the book, autophagy stimulation does not require you to starve yourself. There is a huge difference between starvation and fasting.

On the cellular level, you do want to "starve" your cells, so they enter autophagy mode. But if you are not eating the right foods when you are not fasting, you might get sick when you are fasting. Activating autophagy will clean out your body and make you healthier.

If you don't feel healthier, start with shorter fasts, and build up to longer ones. The art of autophagy is about finding a balance between periods of eating and fasting.

Overdoing autophagy will lead to muscle loss since it breaks down tissue, but you can avoid this by paying attention to your own body and making sure you never get to be an unsafe level of underweight.

When I tell you general tips about autophagy, don't lose sight of your own health metrics and goals. We discuss autophagy in the most generalizable way possible so that anyone can get the most benefit from autophagy. However, autophagy still works on a case-by-case basis.

For instance, if you are more on the leaner side, you should be careful about fasting for too long. Since you have less muscle mass, to begin with, you have to be extra cautious about losing too much from fasting.

A larger person will be able to better get away with fasting for days at a time since they have more muscle mass available to lose without harming their health.

It is hard to generalize how long you should be fasting. It depends on your body size and other factors, which is why you need to speak with your doctor.

Still, your muscle mass is a way to tell if you are going through autophagy for too long or not enough. If you start to look pale and your ribs are sticking out, you are taking autophagy too far. You should never get to this point if you follow this book's guidance.

When deciding how long you should fast, it's important to consider all aspects of your health profile. You need to think about your weight, age, your health history, and how active or sedentary you are. Autophagy is very tissue- and organ-specific, so you have to think about what your health goals are.

If you have heart, liver, or lung problems, you will likely want to avoid water fast because of the strain it puts on your body. But this doesn't mean you have to give up on fasts altogether. You can do a less intense fast, such as an intermittent fast, and still stimulate autophagy.

Intermittent fasting is not recommended for kids and adolescents. People at these ages are still at important times of growth, so they should not be fasting at all. Fasting for autophagy is also not recommended for pregnant women or anyone with heart or liver problems, as it may put too much stress on your body. If you have health concerns, you should only fast if you know your body can handle it.

People with eating disorders should also not fast. Fasting will get you off of your healthy eating patterns, so despite the health benefits, you should hold off on fasting until you no longer struggle with an eating disorder. The same goes for people with diabetes. The balance of insulin in the body of someone with diabetes is too fragile for a diabetic person, so you shouldn't risk fasting.

Chapter 10: The Mental Side

It will be easy to fall out of your autophagy-activation routine if you don't have a well-defined purpose for doing it. Ask yourself why you want to do it in the first place. Is it because you want to be healthier? Look younger? Live longer?

Autophagy will accomplish all of these things. When you are fasting and are really struggling to resist getting a snack, remember your purpose for changing your lifestyle around autophagy.

It is pretty common for people to get excited about changing their life, only to lose interest once the novelty has worn off, and they realize how much they really need to change. You will be no exception to this. You have to plan for this. What are you going to tell yourself to stop from falling out of your routine fasts and keto diet?

The first step to overcoming this barrier is something you have already done. The first step is to believe that autophagy is a good and natural way to keep you healthy and youthful. After coming this far, you have undoubtedly done the first step already.

There is only one more step in the mental aspect of autophagy. This is the step of consistency. Once you get into the habit of your fasting routine and eating healthy autophagy-boosting foods, it will just feel normal to keep living like that.

Psychologists tell us that it takes about one to two months to make a new habit. If you can't do it for a month, that is OK. Start from the beginning and try to go for a month again. It will get easier every time you try it. After you have already done it for a month, you will have already established the routines and small habits necessary to keep activating autophagy.

Remember that eating anything at all will activate mTOR, turning off autophagy, and making the whole day of fasting completely pointless. Once you are in the habit of fasting regularly, it will just seem normal, and the early days of struggling to do it will seem far away.

There are many things that make the autophagy-centered lifestyle different from other health practices. One of them is the simplicity of doing it. When you follow the keto diet, the only things you need to pay attention to on the nutritional label are carbohydrates and the kinds of fats. Compared to other diets, this requires very little of you.

Fasting is even simpler. You don't have to count calories, because you have to stay away from them completely. I'm not saying this is easy, but the hard rule of "don't eat for 24 hours" is very straightforward.

Fasting can be hard for people at first, but you will probably be surprised. People tend to find it to be easier than they expected.

If you fail at your first fast, consider shortening your goal, from 16 hours to 12 hours, for example. There is no rush in developing your fasting routine. When you induce autophagy, you are going the extra mile for your body. Be proud of yourself for that, and let yourself take it slow.

Sometimes the mind can seem like a mystical thing that is impossible to understand, so let's touch briefly on your brain and how it fits into building these new habits.

Much like autophagy, the study of the brain has made great progress in the past decade. Now we know that the cells in your brain (called neurons) are connected to one another with trillions of connections, called synapses.

This is a tremendous discovery. The discovery of synapses tells us that the connections in our brain change constantly, depending on the inputs we give it. If you create new habits like fasting once a week, eating new foods, and exercising regularly, you are creating new connections in your brain. Once these connections have been solidly established (which takes about a month or so, just like a habit), living your life, a new way will just feel normal.

It will be hard as first to follow new routines, but you will get used to it sooner than you think. Soon, they will seem normal, and activating autophagy will be a normal part of your day-to-day life.

Staying in a stress-free environment will really help make your fast a successful one. Don't spend time in environments that may stress you out. Keep people you love around and do activities that you enjoy. You might want to stay at home, so you are close to bed. Sleep will do wonders for the autophagy that you are doing this fast for, so if you want to get extra sleep to pass time during the fast, this is an option.

It is impossible to overstate the importance of decreasing your psychological stress to allow for the best autophagy possible. Do things that relax you and stay away from stressful situations. You can take up yoga or meditation to learn the skill of emptying your mind.

Learning any new habit requires you to change your mental patterns as well as physical ones. Autophagy is no exception. But if you keep reminding yourself your reason for doing it, keep track of your goals and progress in a journal, and stay away from stressful situations, you will be able to succeed in changing your habits.

Write It Down

If you want to keep yourself in check to go through with your fasts, you need to write down your goals somewhere. You need to specify exactly what days you fast and for how many hours. You need to plan what you are going to eat when the fast is over so you can make sure it is healthy.

Write down the time you are allowed to start eating again. Write down how many pounds you want to lose when the fast ends.

You have to keep in mind that you will deal with a lot of emotions when you go through your first fasts. Your emotions will make it a lot harder to keep good track of time, so it is good for you to write down the stipulations for your fast ahead of time and follow them like written instructions.

Writing things down will also help you remember why you are doing the fast in the first place. When you remember you are fasting to lose weight, it will be easier for you to overcome your emotions and continue on with the fast despite them.

You want to start slow with your fasting, but you should still keep your long-term autophagy goals in mind. The best way to think of these goals is in terms of months. The easiest long-term goal to make is: next month; I want to do one 24-hour fast.

Remember that this is a long-term goal. Don't let its seeming difficulty scare you from making achieving smaller goals on the way there. Once you reach this point, don't add to the length of the fast, but add one more fast to the month: next month, I want to do two 24-hour fasts. Going up to 36- and 48-hour fasts may be what you are striving for, but these should be the most distant of your long-term goals.

As we keep saying, consistency is key. The more fasts you do per month, however long or short they are, the closer you are to enjoying the full benefits of autophagy.

How Autophagy Changes Your Brain

The brain is part of our body. Even though we mostly focus on other parts of our body when talking about autophagy, the health of your brain may be even more important.

We sometimes call the brain "the mind," which makes this physical body part seem like it is something other than physical. Once we do away with the mindset that the "mind" is what we want to improve, it starts making a lot more sense that we can make it healthier and work better.

Autophagy will improve the overall health of your body, which includes your brain. With your brain in better shape, it will even be easier to change your habits and activate autophagy, because you will be able to think more clearly. You know that the practices in this book will help put you in better shape, so why wouldn't you want to change your habits to accomplish this?

You will get many of the same health benefits from intermittent and consecutive day fasting as you will from extended water fasting, but you won't get the same spiritual and mental fulfillment. A lot of people who made fasting a part of their daily routine can't imagine their lives without it anymore.

When your body faces a shortage of energy through caloric restriction or fasting, you promote the fusion of mitochondria. As a result, your body's energy demands are decreased because your organelles are healthier and better connected. It also makes you recycle the damaged organelles that used to slow down your cells and make them less efficient. Since autophagy doesn't simply dispose of the organelles and recycles them, the result is more energy for your body that you didn't even know that you had.

This is a book about health and biology, not about the environment, but we can compare the way we think about recycling to the recycling our body does with autophagy, and it will help us think about how this helps our bodies and brains. We say that we "throw things away" when we put them in a trash, and this phrase seems to imply that the garbage is going to be no more. But we all know this is not the case: the garbage adds to a pile of trash in a landfill. It is "away" in the sense that we don't see it, but the garbage is still there.

In our cells, the situation is no different. The cellular garbage is still there whether we like it or not, and we are only adding more to it by eating constantly and never fasting to stimulate autophagy. The methods that promote and stimulate autophagy will take care of this trash, and in our brains, this is even more beneficial.

All of us experience brain fog and a lack of mental clarity from time to time, and when we take care of the cellular garbage in our neurons, we are getting rid of the damaged organelles and misfolded proteins that are making it harder to think.

Getting rid of this waste and making good use of it is even more important in our mitochondria, the most important organelle in all our cells. The key to keeping mitochondria healthy is to maintain energy homeostasis and remove dysfunctional cellular components that are causing inflammation. Time-controlled fasting prevents mitochondrial aging and deterioration. It can also promote the longevity of mitochondria by eliminating the production of reactive oxygen species and free radicals by dysfunctional organelles.

Mitochondrial biogenesis sis the process of building new mitochondria through the activities of certain metabolic regulators.

The key to increased mitochondrial biogenesis and longevity is to prime the body towards a fat burning metabolism. Autophagy activation and the keto diet alike help us achieve this. A fat-burning metabolism increases the ability of your cells to produce energy from its own internal resources (through autophagy), and it also lowers insulin levels (which makes autophagy easier to stimulate later).

Part of what makes fasting so effective is that your body loses the ability to eat as much as it used to. During your fasts, it gets used to having less food, and eating a lot of extra food doesn't feel natural anymore. Long-term water-fasting, in particular, makes people have the epiphany that their body doesn't need as much food as their hunger leads them to believe. It causes you to rethink hunger and what it actually means.

Even if you don't get as many of the benefits that you wanted from your first water fast, you will be sure to get many mental benefits from it. The mental benefits can even outweigh the physical ones. Fasting changes the way that you perceive your relationship with food.

We are so used to being able to eat whenever we want in the developed world. Part of our changed mindset will be a mindset of gratefulness. When you are done fasting and get back to your diet of autophagy-boosting foods and a keto diet (if you are following one), I hope that your time fasting helps you think about how good you have it. You may have problems in your personal life or stresses at work and home, but you should take more time to be happy with what you do have. You have running water and food in the kitchen.

It might seem strange to be grateful for these things, because they are part of your normal life, and everyone you know has these things. But not everyone in the world gets to live a life without thinking about food and water. When you fast, you have a better understanding of these things that we tend to take for granted.

When you are water fasting for just 24 hours, as long as you are a person with a healthy heart and liver, there is no real health risk for fasting for this length of time. In the book, we have called on you to try the 24-hour water fast partly because it is a privilege to be able to see this as a fast and not as a part of normal life. Even if you don't think of the people alive now who aren't able to eat every day, before mass agriculture became a phenomenon, our ancestors did not expect to eat every day either. Autophagy was a normal part of their lives, and they did not have to intentionally fast to get there, because it was normal not to eat every day. Fasting will help put you into this frame of mind, and it will make you more thankful for all the things that you have.

Fasting changes how you eat even if you only fast a few times a month. It makes you think about how important food is in your life. Hopefully, this book has given you some ideas about some nutrients that you should make a part of your diet because a lot of people today spend just twenty minutes or less eating so they can get back to work. But food is something that should be savored, not rushed.

A lot of us don't even realize that we are rushing through our meals because it is part of our normal routine. Besides the mental aspect of how rushing through eating affects us, it has dire health consequences as well. When you rush through your meals, you are not thinking about what it is you are putting into your body.

The keto diet and autophagy together will change how you think about what you put in your body. What you really get from your foods are the nutrients that are in them. These nutrients make everything that your body does possible. Without them, you can miss out on the potential of your brain and body.

By fasting, you think more about your food when you do eat. When you are knowledgeable about the nutrients that are in the food, and you fast, you think a lot about how food will affect your body. Before fasting, you might just eat snack foods without even thinking about it. After fasting, you realize how much harm it would do to your body in the short term, and you also think about how much it is going to disrupt your fast.

Remember, eating carbs and sugary foods makes it a lot harder for your body to start autophagy and ketosis. If you are eating a lot of unhealthy foods, you are making your body take longer to get to your goal of inducing autophagy.

Autophagy doesn't work like other diets because we can't just take "cheat days" where we eat whatever we want. Autophagy requires us to change the habits we have developed throughout our lives so that we don't suppress autophagy. It might not seem like it changes anything if you eat snack foods and other unhealthy foods every once in a while, but long-term consequences aren't always easy to see in the present. You are making it much harder for your body to get into autophagy by eating unhealthy foods. These consequences of unhealthy foods may be even worse than the effects they have on your body. If you keep putting bad foods in your body, your cells will use their energy breaking them down instead of healthier sources of food.

Going through fasts for a long period of time will also give you a clearer mind. The keto diet alone will release ketones into your brain after a very short period of time. Many people who go through long-term fasts say that they feel they can think better and that they feel smarter after fasting. It should make you want to fast to experience what this would be like for you. No one likes to feel foggy in the head — if you are working through a difficult problem in your life, even if the health benefits of fasting are secondary to you, it would be worth it to try a 24-hour water fast and see if it helps you think.

Thinking is at the core of everything we do. As adults, we have well-developed prefrontal cortexes that help us make decisions.

The most important reason that we keep advising you to try the 24-hour hour fast is that, without giving you any serious health risks or requiring a lot of planning, a 24-hour fast will help you think. When you are able to use your brain more effectively, it will make you realize how much better you would feel if you followed a healthy diet, and you incorporated the other ideas in this book that will make you live a healthier life.

The reason we tend to put things off is because of the uncertainty. You might think you will be fine putting off your water fast now; you might be considering it, but you think it would be fine if you did it later. But if you could see yourself in the future after you did your first water fast, you would tell yourself that you should have done it earlier. It will help you think about your health more seriously and push you to prioritize your health in all aspects of your life.

You have this book to look to for help if you don't know where to start. We will be here for you every step of the way. Some of the information we give you may be a lot to take in when you are first getting started, but the good news is you don't have to understand it all at once. We are reaching the end of the book, so you must take your health pretty seriously. You have the tools you need to make a huge difference in it, so the first two things you need to do now are very straightforward. Find a journal where you are going to write down your first specific goal, and look at a calendar to decide what day you will do your 24-hour water fast.

Conclusion

Thank you for making it through to the end of *Book Title*, let's hope it was informative and able to provide you with all of the tools you need to achieve your goals whatever they may be.

Research on the importance of autophagy on our overall health is at the cutting edge of science. Biologists are still trying to learn more about its role in disease prevention, but we already know that autophagy fights off infections and maintains the health of your cells.

This means you can improve your general health by starting with the building blocks that make all that you do possible — your cells.

You've learned there are multiple ways to go about inducing autophagy in your body. The most important are exercising for thirty minutes every day, getting high-quality sleep every night, and, most important of all, getting into a routine of fasting regularly. You will not regret making these life choices.

You know your different options for fasting, and you can choose the one that best suits your own routine and biomarkers. If you are relatively young and healthy, you might be satisfied with doing a 24-hour fast a few times a week.

If you're a little older, you might be looking to kick autophagy into high-gear. You can unleash the full potential of autophagy by doing prolonged water fasts. The research indicates that the number of autophagosomes in your body caps after about 36 hours of fasting. But if you fast for more hours than that, the stress that fasting puts on your body will keep it in the state of autophagy for even longer.

Talk to your doctor about fasting and ask them how much your body can handle. The longer you go, the more your cells will clear out misfolded proteins and toxins. But don't forget about the importance of balance in activating autophagy.

The more experience you have with the keto diet and autophagy, the better you'll become at telling the difference between the normal discomfort of fasting and illness. That said, if you follow the guidance in this book, autophagy will make you healthier, not sick. Don't let the discomfort become an excuse for you to end your fasts early.

Execute your new plan of fasting and eating foods that boost autophagy. You will see the effects on your immune system, energy level, skin tone, and more!

Finally, if you found this book useful in any way, an honest review is always appreciated!

www.ingramcontent.com/pod-product-compliance
Lightning Source LLC
Chambersburg PA
CBHW021515120526
44766CB00007B/387